What Men
Really **Want**
in Bed

D0979924

What Men *Really* Want in Bed

The Surprising Secrets Men Wish Women Knew about Sex

CYNTHIA W. GENTRY AND NIMA BADIEY

QUIVER

Text © 2006 by Cynthia W. Gentry and Nima Badiey

First published in the USA in 2006 by
Quiver, a member of
Quayside Publishing Group
33 Commercial Street
Gloucester, MA 01930

All rights reserved. No part of this book may be reproduced or
utilized, in any form or by any means, electronic or mechanical, without
prior permission in writing from the publisher.

09 08 07 06   1 2 3 4 5

ISBN-13: 978-1-59233-205-2
ISBN-10: 1-59233-205-6

Library of Congress Cataloging-in-Publication Data available

Cover design by Mary Ann Smith
Book design by Leslie Haimes

Printed and bound in USA

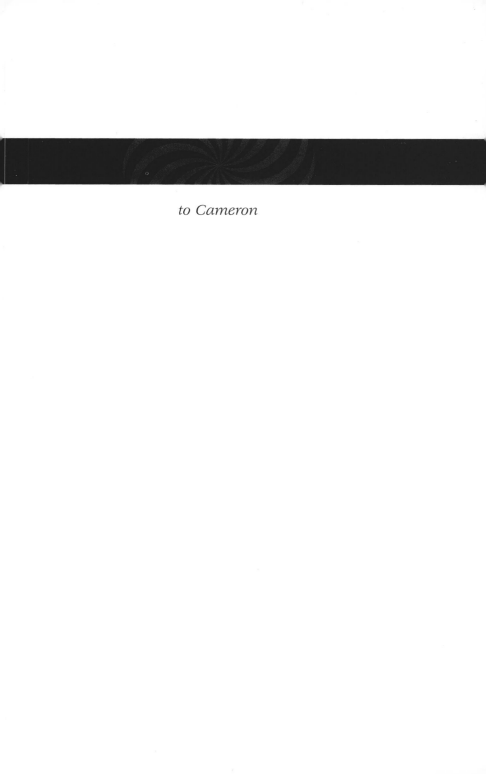

to Cameron

Table of Contents

1. What Do Men Really Want in Bed?   9

2. Secrets of Seduction   15

3. Foreplay Favorites   41

4. Mouth Work   65

5. Handy Maneuvers   93

6. The Main Course   111

7. After the Deed   149

8. Fantasy Island   167

9. How to Find Out What Your Man
   Wants in Bed   195

   Acknowledgments   204

   About the Authors   205

   Index   206

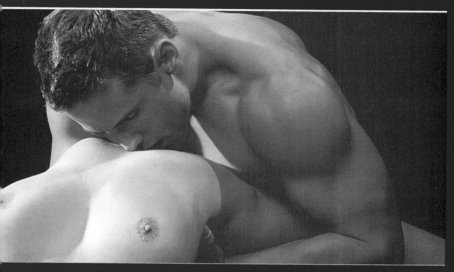

CHAPTER ONE

What <u>Do</u> Men Really Want in Bed?

Ask Them! (We Did.)

Take a quick glance at the "sex instruction" section
of any bookstore. You'll find that most of the books
are written by women, many of whom have

Hi, this is Nima, your copilot on this journey. I'm the "talking head" in this book, occasionally popping up to add a few little nuggets of specifically male wisdom. Since I'm the guy in this relationship, none of my answers will be based on survey data or quantifiable fact, just my own totally biased and usually incorrect opinions. But hey, that's me ... the guy.

■ ■ ■ ■ ■

advanced degrees. You'll find advice on everything from how to perform "mind-blowing" fellatio to how to have an orgasm in less than five minutes. Read *my* book, these experts promise, and you'll be ready to give any guy the night of his life. One popular book even guarantees several hundred "advanced techniques" for "driving a man wild in bed." (We think we'd be exhausted after *five* techniques, much less several hundred, but that's us.)

But in all these rows of books, there's one voice missing. An actual guy's.

Getting frank advice from other women—whether or not they're experts—is fine. But what does your average, lusty, non-Ph.D.-toting man want in bed? Does he really need hundreds of advanced techniques, or does he just want you to show up wearing nothing but a smile? With this book, we set out to answer those questions. We wanted to finally give men a chance to share their real sexual likes and dislikes. Who better than a man to discuss his own sexuality? The idea came out of Cynthia's experience writing *The Bedside Orgasm Book*. As part of her research for the book, she e-mailed several male friends and asked them to share the most exciting thing that a lover had ever done for them in bed. She also asked them how their partners made them feel special and appreciated. Their candid answers showed her that there's an untapped reservoir of information lying in bed next to us women—we're often just too shy, or even too uncomfortable, to ask. Or we might even be *too* comfortable with our partner. In a long-term relationship, it's all too easy to get complacent and forget to check in with each other once in a while.

▋ Getting in Touch with Guys

So, for this book, we broadened our net. Using the site Zoomerang.com, we created an online survey that asked guys to talk about what they wish their wives and girl-friends knew about seduction, foreplay, oral sex, masturbation, intercourse, sexual positions, body image, and more.

A few caveats before we go any further. This was *not* a scientific survey by any stretch of the imagination. Neither of us are sociologists or even scientists (unless you count Nima's background in mechanical engineering, which does, come to think of it, concern how things fit together). The Kinseys, we're not. We're just average people who have an above-average curiosity about sex. We asked the questions to which *we* wanted to know the answers.

We sent the survey to as many guys as we knew, and encouraged them to forward it to their friends. We also sent the survey to several dozen women, asking them to forward it to their husbands, boyfriends, and male friends. In the end, the survey reached nearly 300 men all over the United States, and some in other parts of the world as well. They ranged in age from 23 to 64. They were students, architects, electricians, political activists, scientists, and nurses. But we didn't ask for more demographic information than that, so there's no way to compare a Californian's opinion about oral sex to a Frenchman's. Some men chose to respond anonymously; others created pseudonyms; still others had no problem responding with their own names.

Their answers gave us a fascinating glimpse into the male psyche. Sometimes, we were surprised. We wouldn't have guessed, for instance, that men would rate buttocks over breasts as the sexiest part of a woman's anatomy. Other results confirmed what we already suspected: That most men are nice human beings (duh) who really do want their partners to enjoy themselves during sex—and who will do what it takes to ensure that they do. In return, all they ask is that you show a little enthusiasm. And that you *tell* them what you want, instead of expecting them to read your mind.

Writing this book confirmed our belief that most of our relationship problems could be solved if we just talked to our partners, instead of taking polls of our friends or comparing ourselves to the people we read about in magazines. We hope that *What Men Really Want in Bed* will start that conversation, and get women and their lovers talking to each other.

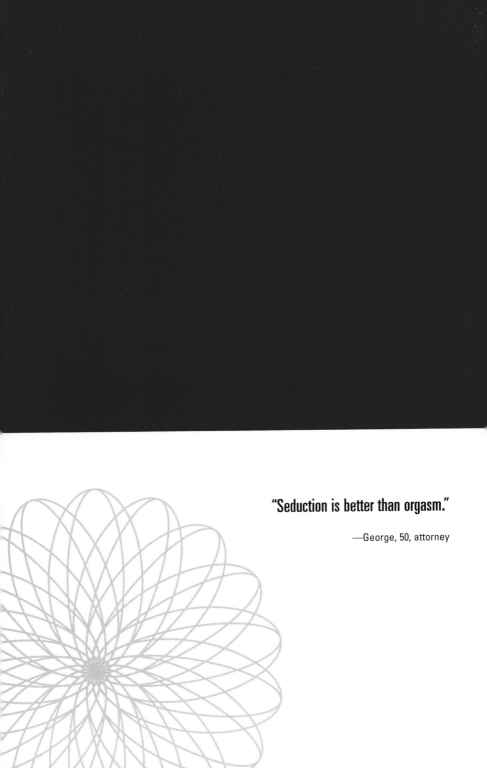

"Seduction is better than orgasm."

—George, 50, attorney

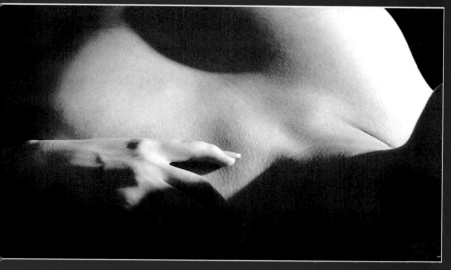

CHAPTER TWO

Secrets of Seduction

Maybe you've just laid eyes on each other across a crowded room. Maybe it's your third date. Maybe you're married! Wherever you are in your relationship, how do you know if he's interested in getting you into bed (hint: he probably is), or just flirting? And how do you show him you want to get frisky, whether he's your husband glued to his computer, or that sexy guy you just met?

We asked guys what they wish women knew about the age-old art of "seduction"—what they wish women knew about how men try to get them into bed. But we also asked them how they like to be seduced. Because, as we found out, men love it when you make the moves. And as more than one man pointed out to us, seduction is a two-way street!

What Men Wish Women Knew about Seduction

If you think men enjoy seduction, you're right. And then some. Here's what our survey told us:

TIP #1: **Men (well, almost all men) are always trying to seduce you**

Most men think about sex constantly. That means that if they're attracted to you, they're probably trying to get you into bed (take it as a compliment), and they'll try almost any means to do it.

It doesn't mean they're bad people. It just means they're horny.

"Men always want to have sex," says Randy, a 45-year-old teacher. "If they show any signs of attraction or interest—or lack of clear disinterest—they're trying to get you into bed."

Some men were even blunter: "If I'm being really nice, I want to sleep with you," states Rob, 45, a self-employed consultant.

Morgan, a 27-year-old financial analyst, agrees. "Know that almost any interaction whatsoever is designed to get you into bed," he says, "and at some level, you should understand this. Only one guy in 1,000 really wants to take you home to 'talk.'"

Keep that in the back of your mind next time some man bares his soul to you. "Any straight man speaking glibly about his emotions is trying to seduce you," says Simon, 36, a software programmer. (Note the word *glib*. Men aren't, as a rule, brought up to discuss their emotions, so if he starts opening up to you after you've known each other a while, that's probably a good sign. But if it's the first date, we'd recommend considering that a flashing yellow light.)

Don't think that he's going to wait until the sun goes down to make his moves. "Asking you to lunch or a casual cup of coffee is actually an invitation for afternoon sex," says Rob, a 36-year-old sales manager.

Some guys use nonverbal cues to indicate their interest. Is he touching you quickly on your arm, shoulder, or back? Maybe grazing your thigh with his fingertips? That's a good sign he's interested in something more than a rousing game of Scrabble.

"Men reflect the stimuli they induce upon their woman," says Clay, a 31-year-old animal control officer. "When I touch my woman seductively, I feel the identical sensation as if she were touching me the same way. So by doing this, I'm hoping to set off a circle of uncontrolled spontaneity."

And be aware that on some level men expect you to *know* that they're trying to seduce you. "Women know we're full of shit," says Ron, a 29-year-old graduate student. But isn't that what makes the dance so much fun?

TIP #2: **A hard-to-get woman is only fun for so long**

No matter how determined they are to get you into bed, don't think that men expect to get lucky right away. For many men, part of what makes seduction so arousing is the delicious thrill of uncertainty. "The chase is often as exciting as the capture," notes Allen, 35, a film producer.

That doesn't mean you should resist his overtures forever—if you're really interested in him. "Hard to get is boring; playful resistance is exciting," says 39-year-old Robert, an attorney. "The hunt is only exciting if the dog eventually catches the fox. If the fox gets away, it's just a lot of running around."

So don't be afraid to show some interest back. "Men are always looking for signs that the woman is interested in sex," says Walt, a 27-year-old marketing manager, "so a woman should be sure to let the man know that she's getting turned on." Most men don't like wasting their time in futile pursuits (if they do, they probably have issues you don't want to deal with); play hard to get for too long, and you may risk ending the chase before you get to be caught.

"Men feel they have to be indirect, but they don't like to play games," states Nigel, a 31-year-old scientist. "If a man is expressing interest, he wants you, period, and usually if he doesn't get clear signals back, he won't proceed."

The key is knowing that seduction involves a certain

SHE SAYS

I hate, hate, hate the expression "hard to get"! If you want to sleep with a guy on the night you meet him or the first date, do it! Just be safe, and don't expect a relationship. (Imagine how pleasantly surprised you'll be if he does call you.) If you decide not to go to bed with him right away, do it because you want to protect yourself emotionally, not because you're trying some lame strategy for hooking him.

■ ■ ■ ■ ■

amount of playfulness. "We test the waters with our flirting to see how you react," comments Ben, a 40-year-old architect. "If you're offended by comments like 'you have great legs' or 'you've got a cute tush,' then we aren't going to try to seduce you. Lighten up!"

TIP #3: **Seducing a woman Is harder than it looks**

TIP #3A: **Men are human, too**

HE SAYS

Men are simple. I admit that freely. We don't understand calls that go unreturned, or "I'll call you later" blow-offs. Closure is as much for us as it is for you, but in the light of uncertainty, we're more likely to continue pursuing unless there are clear signs that it's futile. Don't be afraid to speak up and express yourself (positively or negatively). Just remember that what goes around comes around, so if you have to shut it down, be definitive, but nice.

■ ■ ■ ■ ■

Girls, have a little compassion for your guy. Yes, men want to seduce you. That does *not* mean, however, that they actually know how to do it. T.J., a 42-year-old musician, says it best: "I wish women knew how hard it is to actually seduce a woman. Every woman responds differently, and yet men are expected to be able to anticipate and adapt."

Guy after guy in our survey confessed to a certain amount of insecurity about their seduction skills:

* "Despite appearances, we're pretty unsure about going to bed with you, too. Give us a readable sign. Leave a graceful out (for either of us) if possible." —Sam, 46, business consultant

* "Most men are clueless about how to seduce a woman." —Mike, 23, restaurant worker/student

* "A lot of men don't know how to get women in bed. It's more that they stumble onto it. Most sincere men are very insecure about seduction. The men who are confident seducers are usually jerks and spoil it for the rest of us." —J.B., 50, software engineer

* "We don't really know what we're doing—humor us." —Rick, 27, student

* "Some guys are just as uncomfortable with their bodies as women are. A lot of times, we just see getting the woman into bed as a chance to celebrate her body." —Jordan, 45, marketing executive

So be a little sensitive to his feelings (refer back to Corollary Tip #3A). If you're not interested in his overtures, don't drag it out. "No one likes rejection, but it's okay to be direct and say thanks but no thanks," advises Marcus, 47. "Just be tactful about it. Instead of not calling or being overly polite, say you're otherwise engaged or just unavailable."

This brings us to our next—and possibly most important—tip about men and seduction:

 TIP #4: Men aren't jerks Yes, men like sex, and they're usually trying to get you to have it with them. But that's *not* to say that every friendly guy you meet is an insincere player with nothing more on his mind than a one-night stand. "They really do like you," advises Pete, a 42-year-old sales representative.

"Most men won't even try employing 'tactics' like one-liners and relying on alcohol," says Jack, a 52-year-old graphic designer. "In fact, most men I know object to the whole idea of manipulating women (or anyone else) to do anything."

Men understand that you need to trust a man before becoming intimate with him. Bruce, a 31-year-old financial planner, speaks for many when he says, "I want to build a trust level first with a woman, so she feels that she can be in bed with me without being uncomfortable."

In fact, the whole idea of seduction for seduction's sake turns many men off. "Not to sound like I'm too caring, but seducing a woman just to get her into bed just doesn't do it for me," says Patrick, a 41-year-old marketing professional. "If I feel a connection while we're kissing, I know that the relationship will eventually end up in the bedroom."

So don't write off that nice guy who doesn't have the smoothest moves. "Men who seem very charming are probably deploying a skill they've learned and therefore are not necessarily good guys, but men who have no skill at seem-

HE SAYS

Sex is more than Tab "A" in Slot "B." We're not assembling IKEA furniture, we're practicing the art of seduction—so it's doubly important to be open about your feelings and desires.

Fun Fact: Men know only 1 percent of what women wish they knew, so if you really want a guy to do something special, you have to let him know. We hear a lot of women gripe that the best men are taken or gay. If you find a great guy, it's okay to "invest" in him. We're not born with all the knowledge we need to be successful with women, but if you put in the time and effort, what you get in return is often orders of magnitude greater. Remember, we're willing to learn if you're willing to teach!

■ ■ ■ ■ ■

HE SAYS

The biggest and nicest surprise you can get is to learn that someone's got the hots for you, especially when you had no idea they were interested. (Of course, it helps if you're interested back.) There's nothing sexier than a woman seducing a man. We love the idea of being wined, dined, and ... stuff. And we even like being on the bottom during sex (it's easier on our backs).

■ ■ ■ ■ ■

ing charming might actually be the only good men in the room," says 35-year-old Richard, a teacher. "It's easier and far more

 TIP #5: **Why give the game away?**

fun to teach a good man to be charming than to teach a charming man to be good."

As candid as most men were about sharing their seduction secrets with us, some guys simply played coy.

"I'm not sure that there's anything in particular that I'd want women to know about this," said one man, who didn't give his name. Another commented, "Why give the game away?"

Are these men such masters of seduction that giving away their methods would completely kill their mojo? Not at all. They simply fall into the school that sees mystery as the key ingredient of the dance between men and women.

"Women don't need to know about how we try to seduce them," says 29-year-old Brian, a filmmaker. "That's why it's so fun to play the game. If they knew the tricks, it wouldn't be as exciting."

Of course, there's one other reason that men were reticent about opening up their seduction tool kit: They figure women are already wise to their tricks. "I'm not sure women need to know any more about how men try to get them in bed," laughs P.B., a 51-year-old corporate headhunter. "They have plenty of experience."

Girls, It's Okay to Make the First Move!

So you get our drift: Men like the thrill of seduction. But that doesn't mean that they always like to do the work. When it comes to getting frisky, do men like women to take the initiative? A whopping 57 percent came back with a resounding "Yes, absolutely!" A substantial number—43 percent—said it depended on the woman and the situation. Not a single man said that he'd prefer to initiate.

One man commented that seductive give-and-take between the sexes is what keeps things interesting: "Women *do* sometimes need to seduce men to keep the balance of sexual tension," says 34-year-old Malcolm, a manager. Dan, a 38-year-old real estate agent, agrees: "Assuming I always wanted to get women into bed, which I don't, I'd say women need to be more comfortable taking the lead."

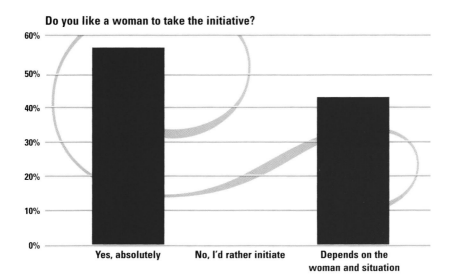

Do you like a woman to take the initiative?

Yes, absolutely	No, I'd rather initiate	Depends on the woman and situation

HE SAYS/SHE SAYS

Nima says: When's the last time a guy said "no" to sex?!

Cynthia responds: Uh, wishful thinking, honey. Believe it or not, it does happen. Don't try to hop on your guy during the crucial last few minutes of the championship game, or when he's stressed or simply exhausted. Repeat it like a mantra: "Men are human, too."

■ ■ ■ ■ ■

Not to mention the fact that many men are simply tired of playing seducer. "It's tough for us to initiate every move," complains Paul, a 29-year-old graduate student. "Why can't it be the other way around once in a while?"

How to Seduce a Man

So, given that men *want* you to seduce them every once in a while, what's the sexiest move or gesture you can make to signal your interest? Here are some tips from men on how *they* like to be seduced:

TIP #1: **Be direct**

News flash: Men can't read minds. In fact, Cynthia says she's never yet met a man with ESP, despite her claims that Nima should "just know" when she wants him to take out the gar-bage. Don't be so coy that he can't tell whether or not you're interested. "Cut to the chase," advises Sam, a 52-year-old musician, a sentiment echoed by a majority of guys in our survey.

"If a woman wants to be with me, she should just come out and say it," agrees David, 43, a systems administrator.

"I *like* a girl to tell me she's interested," production assistant Ted, 27, assures us.

And when some men say "be direct," they mean it. For Nigel, "an explicit come-on" is the best way to seduce him. Another man advises a woman to "do the same thing I'd do to her: get me drunk, tell me I'm hot, and start touching my breasts." Alex, a 32-year-old operations manager, likes "a look and being led to the bedroom, living room, or even the car!"

TIP #2: **Be real** Along with wanting you to be direct, men in our survey say they want you to be yourself, because they find nothing more off-putting than someone trying to play a part. "Being real is so much sexier than trying to play at being a femme fatale or ice queen," advises Patrick, a 40-year-old writer. "A smile in your eyes is sexier than trying to be cold and sultry."

"I like it if she verbalizes what she wants and is confident in her sexuality," says William, 39, a business development manager. "I want to know she's not just along for the ride (figuratively and literally)."

TIP #3: **Get physical** The number-one indication a guy has that you want to get physical is when you get ... well, physical. There's nothing that signals your desire to a man better than touch, subtle or otherwise.

"I know she's interested when she starts to be 'touchy feely' with me," says Bruce. "It turns me on when a woman starts touching my arm or shoulders in public. It's usually a good sign."

For some men, a gentle or supposedly "innocent" touch is all it takes. Any of the following gestures can signal your interest:

* "Kissing my neck."
 —Sam, 52, musician

HE SAYS

Ask and ye shall receive sex. Drop hints, and you'll probably get nothing. If you can't speak up for yourself, you won't get the wall-pounding, sheet-ruffling, ear-splitting orgasm you so richly deserve.

■ ■ ■ ■ ■

* "Playful conversation punctuated by little touches."
  —Patrick, 40, writer

* "Eye contact, light touches." —Claude, 34, musician

* "Playfulness that includes little touches anywhere on my body, especially my neck." —Sam, 46, business consultant

* "Gentle, subtle body contact. Perhaps a hand against the side of my hand." —Dan, 38, real estate agent

* "With intention, her hand on my arm."
  —Ralph, 34, graduate student

* "A gentle or subtle grab of my leg or my arm."
  —Scott, 29, student

* "Supple body movement—light, casual touching. Brushing her breasts against me." —George, 50, attorney

  Other guys get turned on by more aggressive moves. He's not getting the point? Try one of these:

* "Strong hug and a French kiss, or a wink and a smile followed by licking your lips." —Name withheld

* "A juicy French kiss and a genital caress."
  —Randy, 45, teacher

* "Rub against me—or reach out for a kiss."
  —Joe, 59, consultant

* "Rub my inner thigh." —Peter, 58, nurse

* "Grab my ass or give my crotch a playful squeeze! Straddle me with your clothes on and kiss me." —Ben, 40, architect

* "One time my girlfriend licked her lips, grabbed my shirt, and pulled me into the bedroom. That was hot."
  —Jordan, 45, marketing executive

But no matter how many times you "accidentally" brush against him, remember that eventually, you may have to speak up. "First, if she finds any excuse to physically touch me repeatedly, that is a sure and sexy sign of interest, but she will never close the deal unless she gets frank about what she wants or likes," says Richard.

COROLLARY TIP #3A: Don't forget about the rest of his body

Sure, some men like you to go right for their package. But don't limit your seduction moves to blatant grabs for what's between his legs, or you may miss out on a chance to truly drive him wild. "Men are not just their penises," admonishes William, 39. "Don't be so focused there. Pay attention to our whole body. It's covered in erogenous zones."

TIP #4: It's in the eyes

Don't underestimate the power that your eyes have. Over and over, the men in our survey cited "eye contact" as the surest signal they can get that a woman is trying to seduce them. Your gaze can be quick, constant, or out-and-out direct. "Do me with your eyes and be obvious about it," advises Brian, the 29-year-old filmmaker. Here are some other tips:

* "Look in my direction and then toward the bedroom."
  —Jeffrey, 51 (no profession given)

* "Give me a lingering look, a sexy smile, and a slow lean into my ear to tell me something."
  —Ted, 44, logistics manager

HE SAYS/SHE SAYS

Nima says: Here's another tip. Play with your food ... seductively. If a guy doesn't understand that you want sex as you suck on that asparagus or deep-throat the banana, then he's a wanker.

Cynthia responds: As you might guess, this technique only works well if you're lucky enough to be with a man who has an oral fixation.

■ ■ ■ ■ ■

* "Make direct eye contact without B.S. conversation, and acknowledge our attraction."
—Allen, 35, film producer

You don't have to make campy goo-goo eyes to get your point across. "Mischievous looks work for me," says Matt, a 46-year-old political activist. "Think sly, versus brazen. Too over-the-top makes me laugh."

 TIP #5: **Talk to him**

Some men respond best to verbal cues. "You can't beat a woman walking up to you and striking up a conversation," says Paul, 29. Suggestions for engaging in the art of verbal seduction include:

* "Initiate a conversation and maintain it."
—Steve, 27, student

* "Talk dirty. An indiscreet comment goes a long way."
—Tom, 31, attorney

* "Show sexual wit without undue bluntness."
—Robert, 39, attorney

* "Whisper to me. Give me compliments."
—Matt, 46, political activist

* "Engage me in unexpectedly frank conversation. It doesn't even have to be about sex."
—Simon, 36, programmer

The element of surprise can also rev up a guy's engine. So get his imagination running when he least expects it, and he'll be panting with anticipation. "Allude to sex while in a nonsexual situation, like during lunch or on the phone," suggests Patrick, 41. "Telling me what you like or what you'd like to do to me later—and knowing that we're both thinking about it until we actually get together—tends to make for some intense sessions."

 TIP #6: **Have fun!** If you're going to take the sexual initiative, for God's sake, enjoy yourself. Sex is supposed to be fun, not a battle. Nothing's sexier than a woman who honestly likes sex.

"Men like to be seduced by women who like to be seduced themselves," says Gene, a 64-year-old writer. "A woman who makes it clear she does not want to participate in her own seduction is not going to seduce anyone herself. It's an interactive process, not a one-way street."

What Part of Your Body Does He Find Sexiest?

When it comes to seducing a man, what part of your body does he focus on? A majority of men—25 percent—said it's your tush. We delved a little deeper to find out why:

* "Skin is sexy, curves are sexy. The butt has them both. Also, even when a woman is practically nude, there is usually something covering part of it, even if it is just a

G-string. Therefore, anytime you get to see it completely uncovered, it is very erotic."
—David, 43, systems administrator

* "Generally, if a woman takes even halfway decent care of herself, she has a nice tush. That, or Levi Strauss is to blame. Because there's nothing better than watching your woman walk across a room while she's wearing her favorite pair of jeans."
—Patrick, 41, marketing professional

* "For whatever reason, curves are sexy. In addition to this, the tush is a naughty spot."
—Mike, 23, restaurant worker/student

* "I think the 'tush' says a lot about a woman as well as being the part that completes the curviness of a woman's body (when viewed top to bottom) for me. The tush is one of my first clues about how active or athletic a woman is, and how she takes care of herself." —George, 50, attorney

* "I think because it is one part that is utilized during sex (to grab onto and get some traction) and visually appealing to boot." —Andy, 45, electrician

* "I guess it goes with my favorite position, doggy style. I'm not sure I can explain it; it's more instinctive than intellectual. To me a woman's tush is the embodiment of her sexuality, the complex curves and secret entryway to her inner sanctum." —Jay, 50, software engineer

* "A nice butt looks great no matter what you're wearing, and I think we're hardwired to target it. You just can't look at a

nice butt without thinking of sex."

—Patrick, 40, writer

* "It's a primal instinct that goes back to the caveman days when the gals were always running away from us ... as we chased them down, literally. It was the natural thing to keep focused on." —Rob, 36, salesman

When they refer to primal instinct and hardwiring, Rob and Patrick may be on to something. We asked Stanford anthropologist Dr. Timothy King why the female buttocks would be so attractive to men.

HE SAYS/SHE SAYS

Nima says: The term "ass-man" can either be a derogatory moniker or a label of distinction. Men see it as the latter. But we like all parts of you. If a woman has a fine ass ... or breasts ... or legs ... or eyes ... or lips ... then it's our duty to acknowledge and worship it.

Cynthia responds: And don't think that a "fine ass" equals an airbrushed model ass like you see in magazines. I've always been conscious of having what I consider a substantial derriere, but Nima can't seem to keep his hands off my butt, whether I'm a size 6 (now a distant memory) or a size 12 (pregnancy). Makes me think that there's something to that "waist-to-hip" ratio/fertility thing.

■ ■ ■ ■ ■

"The butt is not actually just the butt—it represents the ass-to-waist ratio, or the 'degree of hips,'" Dr. King says. "A butt of a certain size is a demonstration of fitness, or a caloric intake healthy enough to have kids, and waist-to-hip ratio indicates a birth canal wide enough to sufficiently handle birthing." (In fact, underweight women who are having trouble getting pregnant are often advised to gain weight, as a too-low body fat ratio can negatively affect fertility, as can, on the other end of the scale, obesity.) While this doesn't explain the attraction some men have for stick-figure-like supermodels, it does provide some food for thought about the age-old subconscious urges that motivate us. (Discuss among yourselves.)

So if he's *not* looking at your butt, what else does he notice? Not surprisingly, given how men like you to seduce them, the eyes had it next, with 14 percent picking your peepers as the physical feature that draws them in. "The eyes are the window to the booty," says Andy, 45. "They tell you if you're going to get some. I pay attention to them at all times."

Somewhat to our surprise, given our culture, breasts came in third place. "Breasts are also curvy and naughty, like buttocks," says Mike, 23. "They are soft yet firm, vary significantly from woman to woman, and are an erogenous zone. You can often see part of them (cleavage) but not all, which drives your imagination wild."

A few men picked shoulders. "I said shoulders because I love the very feminine lines starting from the neck, down the nape, and across the shoulder," says Paul. "Plus, unlike the buttocks, breasts, or other body parts, shoulders are always 'out there' to appreciate, touch, and kiss."

Some men zeroed right in on the genitals. "I think anyone who has gone down on a woman, and enjoys it, knows why men are so infatuated with that area of a woman," muses Patrick, 41. "The smell. The texture. The taste. The way it swells and gets wet when it's touched in a way the owner enjoys. Ahhh, the wetness."

But some men refused to pick just one part of the body. "Only one!" protested one man. "You must be joking!"

What female body part do you find the sexiest?

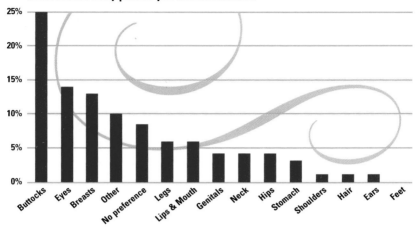

These men take the entire woman—or certain areas—into account. "It's a package deal," says Pete, while T.J. commented that he's attracted to "her whole face, neck, and hair taken together."

Other men say that they find different women sexy for different reasons, while some got more specific. For example, Xavier, a 40-year-old engineer, said that "bare thighs" are what attracted him to women's legs.

HE SAYS

Guys notice everything, even if they pretend not to. When you change your hair, paint your toes, wear outfits that better show off your curves ... we notice all of these things. We're not perverts, just connoisseurs of the finer things in life.

■ ■ ■ ■ ■

No matter what you're wearing, don't forget the sense of smell. Our eyes can perceive up to 256 levels of light, our ears can hear up to 25 kilohertz, and our taste buds can sense four different flavors. But our olfactory senses can identify more than 30,000 different chemicals. Of your five senses, smell is most strongly associated with memory and pheromone response. It's your strongest weapon, so use it.

■ ■ ■ ■ ■

Dressing for Seduction

If you want to get him interested, what's the sexiest outfit you can wear? Men's answers ran the gamut:

* 21 percent said they like revealing "sexy, club-going" outfits.

* 14 percent like casual clothes, like jeans and T-shirts.

* 14 percent are turned on by fancy lingerie, such as lacy bras, panties, and thongs.

* 13 percent love it when you dress up in "classy" outfits like a cocktail dress or evening gown.

* 11 percent simply want to see you in your bare skin!

But a substantial number of men have their own ideas about what kinds of clothes make a woman sexy, ranging from sleeveless shirts to casual sundresses. Jeans make a frequent appearance: "White tank, jeans, bare feet, oh *my*!" gushes Andy, while Patrick, the 41-year-old marketing professional, likes "tight jeans, tight halter top, and a baseball hat."

What's the sexiest outfit a woman can wear to seduce you?

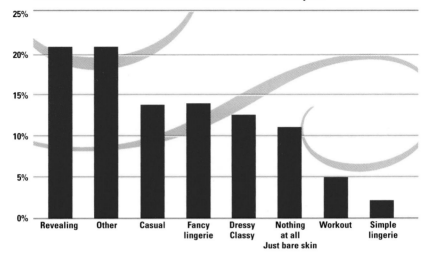

While some men aren't picky ("all of the above," says Brian, a 37-year-old entrepreneur), for some, believe it or not, it's business clothes:

* "Business casual, because I see them in meetings." —Malcolm, 34, manager

* "All of the above! Also women's business clothes." —Patrick, 40, writer

* "Professional attire (skirt, blouse, etc.)." —Richard, 35, teacher

Still others define "sexy" as whatever you feel most comfortable in. "Whatever is most about her essence," says George, 48. "Whatever she can display her confidence in," says Dave, a 41-year-old executive. So if tight pants and revealing tops aren't your thing, don't fret. If *you* feel sexy in what you're wearing, it'll come across.

Will He Respect You in the Morning?

How quickly does a man want to hop into bed after he finds himself attracted to you? The answer may surprise you: For the majority of men, it depends on a variety of factors—but the most important is that elusive ingredient known as "chemistry." The men we surveyed were adamant about its importance.

* "I could find someone very good-looking, but if there's no 'chemistry,' I couldn't care less about having sex with her. The chemical thing is very important because we can't control it; it arises from our comfort level, our genuine attraction, and our respect for the woman. It also is a good indication of a lasting relationship." —Andy, 45, electrician

* "Everything depends on chemistry! If a woman's personality is flat or annoying or awkward, it doesn't matter what she looks like or what she's wearing." —Patrick, 40, writer

* "Chemistry and other factors play a huge role for reasons I don't fully understand. Sometimes I can feel an immediate and strong sexual urge. Other times, it takes a while to develop some attraction." —George, 50, attorney

* "Things in the bedroom, even the first time, are so much more enjoyable when you have a certain comfort level with each other. Several casual dinners. Some back-and-forth banter via e-mail. A couple of phone conversations. All of these things add up quickly and give both people an idea if there's mutual interest/attraction to move the situation to a sexual one. These things can take place in less than a week or over several." —Patrick, 41, marketing professional

* "If she's so annoying, cold-fishy, or bitchy that it bothers me, I'm not going to be interested in performing, even once. If it's someone with whom I feel an immediate and reciprocated connection, I'm not so worried about sealing the deal immediately because I'm sure I'll see her again." —Nigel, 31, scientist

* "There has to be good chemistry if a relationship is to develop. I think about that going into it." —Peter, 58, nurse

* "Chemistry is a lead-in to other aspects of the relationship. Sexuality is just one conduit for communication. Few guys really want to be porno stars. They might want to get laid, but most want some aspect of their relationship with a woman to have some sexual flare. To get that flare going requires chemistry." —Malcolm, 34, manager

Some men are frank about wanting to consummate the relationship quickly. "If I have any interest in her, I will want to sleep with her as soon as possible," says one man. Agrees Rob, the 36-year-old salesman, "I believe it's a fairly normal hormonal urge to want to bed an attractive woman without delay."

But others want to wait, and admit that while the desire to sleep with you may be there, they don't feel compelled to hop into bed right away. "The feeling may be immediate—the action may come later," says George, 48, a marketing consultant.

Adds Paul, 29: "Sometimes it's purely sexual, and you just wanna 'get nekkid' ASAP. Other times you want to take it slower: want to enjoy getting to know them, enjoy the anticipation of what's to come, and hey, maybe you also don't want to go too quick for fear of screwing (no pun

How quickly do you want to "do the deed" after meeting a woman who attracts you?

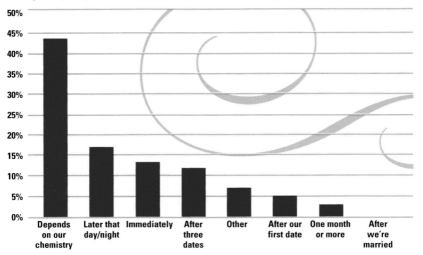

Depends on our chemistry	Later that day/night	Immediately	After three dates	Other	After our first date	One month or more	After we're married

intended!) the whole thing up! There's nothing wrong with a bit of old-fashioned courting and dating."

And although it flies in the face of what we've been led to believe, many men want to postpone the action *because they want to get to know you better.* "I want to wait until after I get to know her and feel comfortable," says David, echoing the sentiments of many men who responded to our survey.

HE SAYS

Let's not be naive here: When a man says he wants to get to know you better, it *does* mean he wants to have sex with you. But that's not a bad thing! For us, sex *is* a way to get to know a woman better. You both expose yourself, literally, and through the very mechanical act of it, you discover an intimacy that wasn't there before. How many times have you confessed a dark or dirty secret to your man while in bed? For us, sex is just a way to cut through all the crap and get to know someone on a totally different plane.

■ ■ ■ ■ ■

The Bottom Line

In the end, any seduction tip comes with one whopper of a caveat: Every man is different. Sure, our survey seems to indicate some general patterns, but remember that what works with one guy may fall flat with another—which is a good argument for getting to know a guy before you pull out your best moves. But be yourself and let him know by look, comment, or touch that you're interested, and you can't go wrong.

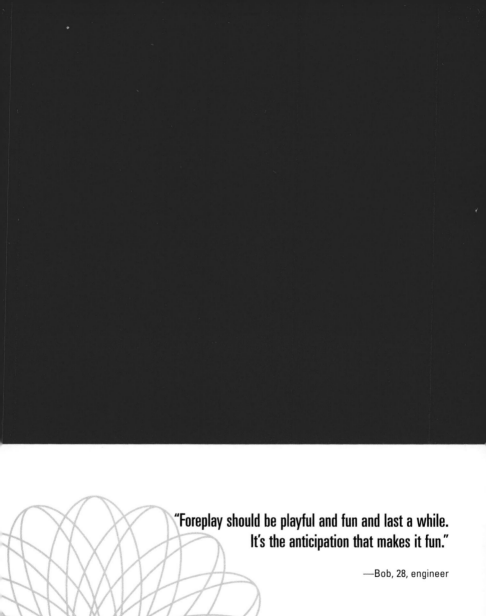

"Foreplay should be playful and fun and last a while.
It's the anticipation that makes it fun."

—Bob, 28, engineer

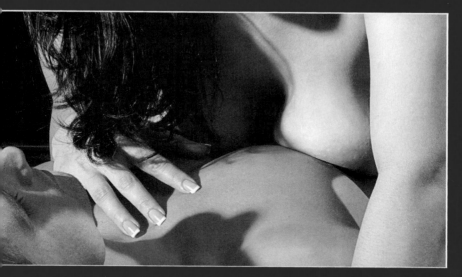

CHAPTER THREE

Foreplay Favorites

There's a lot to be said for passionate, down-and-dirty, "I've got to have you now" sex—the kind where you go at each other like crazed monkeys. But savvy couples know that foreplay can send both parties into a state of crazed anticipation and turn good sex into out-of-this-world love-making. And let's face it, not every woman can go from zero to sixty in ten seconds: Most of us need a little warm-up before we're primed for action. As one of Cynthia's more colorful friends said to her, "You gotta warm up the pan before you put the meat in!"

Many gals worry that their guys don't have the patience to get them where they need to go. Good news: Our survey revealed that just isn't the case. As it turns out, the majority of men love everything leading up to the main event. We asked them what gets them the hottest—and what turns them off before they even get to the bedroom. They also told us the kind of kiss they like, their hottest nongenital erogenous zone, and what sort of down-south grooming turns them on. Read on to find out what they said.

What Men Wish Women Knew about Foreplay

Here you have the truth about men and foreplay—straight from the source.

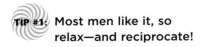 **TIP #1:** Most men like it, so relax—and reciprocate!

First of all, don't feel guilty if you need some time to reach peak arousal. It's physiologically necessary. What's more, we found that the majority of men in our survey are glad to spend a little time getting you warmed up. They want to savor the entire event rather than racing toward the finish line.

"It's not a chore for us—we want to do what turns you on," says Nigel, a 31-year-old scientist, echoing a sentiment expressed by many of the men who responded. So relax and revel in the sensations, because that's what he wants you to do. "Just enjoy yourself," says Luke, a 32-year-old student.

And let him know that you *are* enjoying it! "A 'let's-get-it-over-with' attitude kills everything," Greg, 35, an engineer, points out.

And don't distract yourself by worrying that you'll have to "give back" right away. As it turns out, men like to give (and give and give)! Boris, a 43-year-old creative director, notes that the woman "doesn't always need to reciprocate. It's nice to let her relax and express pleasure without feeling that she needs to give back."

That doesn't mean, however, that when it comes to your guy, you can skip the warm-up, either. The guys we heard from enjoy giving *and* receiving:

* "Guys like foreplay, too. We both know where it's going to finish, so let's take our time." —Patrick, 41, marketing professional

* "I like to be kissed and touched all over, too!" Patrick, —40, writer

* "I wish women knew that the sitcom image of men is crap. Men like foreplay, but it needs to be mutual." —T.J., 42, musician

* "Don't be afraid to get creative or take the initiative. Foreplay is fun." —Mike, 23, restaurant worker/student

* "We like that movie as much as you do, as long as it's clear there's going to be a happy ending." —Simon, 36, programmer

Yes, there were a few men in our survey who deemed foreplay "overrated" and noted that men don't always need it, but they were in the minority.

So don't worry that you're not jumping right to intercourse. Whether you're engaging in sexy talk over dinner or kissing every inch of his body, chances are that he's enjoying every second. "Take your time," advises Pete, a 42-year-old salesman.

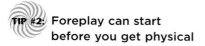

TIP #2: Foreplay can start before you get physical

Before we go any further, let's take a big step back. What exactly qualifies as "foreplay"? The *American Heritage Dictionary* defines it as "sexual stimulation preceding intercourse." But the dictionary doesn't say when, where, and how that stimulation can occur—and we'll tell you right now, it doesn't always have to happen after you have your clothes off. In fact, "it starts far earlier than most women think," asserts Gene, a 64-year-old writer.

As Scott, a 29-year-old graduate student, says: "Foreplay doesn't need to begin in the bedroom. A sexy dance at a club, a playful caress at the movie theater, or a seductive look at a restaurant can be just as effective in building up towards intercourse."

Let's put it this way: Some not-so-innocent flirtation gets your minds racing as you imagine the delights in store. "Sometimes we need a little teasing," says Jordan, a 45-year-old marketing professional. "Good foreplay begins hours ahead of the actual act and builds in intensity throughout the night."

So don't neglect the power of the imagination. A few well-placed words can fire you both up: "The best foreplay is dirty talk," says Bruce, a 31-year-old financial planner, while engineer Xavier, 40, advises women to "seduce with your eyes."

Want more ideas? Refer back to the previous chapter, "Secrets of Seduction," on page 15 for tips on how to get you both in the mood. But don't think you need fancy techniques. Sometimes all it takes is a deep, lingering kiss. Which brings us to our next tip:

Refer back to the previous chapter, "Secrets of Seduction," on page 15

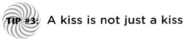 **A kiss is not just a kiss**

HE SAYS

Half the guys I've talked to admit that it's harder to get a girl to kiss them than sleep with them. Maybe that's because kissing is such an intimate act.

■ ■ ■ ■ ■

Here's another thing men want you to know about foreplay: Learn to be a good kisser. "Kissing is key," advises William, a 39-year-old business development executive. "Linger with soft, sensuous kisses for a while to get the mood to the right level. Kissing says everything about who you are in bed. A bad kisser is probably going to be bad in bed."

He wasn't the only man to focus on the power of a good kiss. "Kissing is the best," says Joe, 59, a consultant, summing up an emotion expressed by many men.

 Speak up about what you need

Want to ensure that foreplay does get you ready for action? Well, speak up! Don't expect him to read your mind. "Be more vocal," pleads Sam, a 52-year-old musician. Adds Richard, a 35-year-old teacher, "It's okay to playfully instruct men who don't know what they are doing, and tell them what they *should* be doing."

It may be as easy as letting your man know that you need a little warm-up. Remember, he's built differently than you are. "Men need to learn foreplay's importance for you," counsels Claude, a 54-year-old musician. "Most

HE SAYS

If I had to choose between foreplay and afterplay, I'd choose the foreplay. However, although we enjoy it as much as you do, keep in mind that we probably don't need as much to get our engines going.

■ ■ ■ ■ ■

men don't need it in the same way. We're wired up and ready at the drop of a hat."

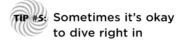

TIP #5: Sometimes it's okay to dive right in

Another important fact about foreplay is this: It's okay to skip it. Like we said, there's absolutely nothing wrong with tear-your-clothes-off, drunken-monkey sex. You and your man may simply not have the time or inclination for hours of luxurious foreplay. As Ben, a 40-year-old architect, says, "Sometimes it's great to skip foreplay all together and just go for it!" (We'd bet that if you get to the point where you just *have* to have each other *now*, the mental foreplay has been going on for some time.)

As with all aspects of sex, you simply need to gauge your partner's mood. "Be responsive," suggests Sam, a 46-year-old business consultant. "Sometimes hours of foreplay are wonderful; other times, a five-minute rush is perfect. There's no best formula." Be in the moment, to put it in Zen terms.

And make sure he knows that you're okay with—that, in fact, you like—the occasional quickie. "The usual rules of reciprocity say we have to 'pay up front' and then we get to enjoy things," says Alex, a 32-year-old manager. "Let us know that isn't always needed."

HE SAYS

Is this a good time to remind everyone of the long-lost art of the "nooner"? If you can swing it, arrange to meet at lunchtime one day. You'll go back to work with a big smile on your faces.

■ ■ ■ ■ ■

TIP #6: **Take your time**

And what about those times when you've got all the time in the world? Know that some guys love long, drawn-out lovemaking sessions. "Make foreplay last," advises P.B., a 51-year-old corporate headhunter.

COROLLARY TIP #6A: **A man is not just his member**

"It's not a sprint, it's a marathon (well, maybe a half-marathon)," adds Rob, 28, an engineer. "Foreplay shouldn't be quick. It should be playful and fun and last a while. It's the anticipation that makes it fun."

The men in our survey want you to know that although they relish an enthusiastic lover, they need finesse as much as you do. Don't simply dive for your partner's nether regions and think that's enough (even though sometimes it might be).

"Men like to be touched, too," says Marcus, 47, a general manager. "Use your hands on our whole bodies, not just our genitals. Find *our* erogenous zones."

In fact, although we said this in chapter 2, it's worth repeating: A man is not just his penis. "Direct stimulation is not always good," says Robert, a 39-year-old attorney. "If you're in the mood, don't just grab my penis like it's some kind of 'on/off' switch."

Ditto, says Ted, 44, a logistics manager. "Please don't expect my penis to leap to immediate attention. Touch me all over."

Ron, a 29-year-old graduate student, puts it more bluntly. "Don't spend too much time working the rod, since that's what's going to be used later." In fact, "too much rubbing can hurt!" says Steve, 27, a waiter.

HE SAYS

The bottom line is that you need to be gentle—but not *too* gentle!

■ ■ ■ ■ ■

That's not to say you should ignore your man's member altogether. "Penile stimulation during foreplay prolongs and intensifies intercourse for both parties," comments J.B., 50, a software engineer. "Women need to be comfortable holding, caressing, and kissing a man's penis. It's not about bringing the man to orgasm; it's more about women finding the same pleasure in stimulating men that men find in stimulating women."

And when you do handle the family jewels, many of our respondents reminded women to take care. "Don't forget lotion or oil when you're rubbing our genitals," says Randy, a 45-year-old teacher.

What Type of Foreplay Gets Men the Hottest?

You get the point: Men like foreplay. But what kind? The answers we got in our survey were as varied as the men who answered, but they fell into a few general categories.

 TIP #1: **Men like mental foreplay**

You've probably heard the saying that "99 percent of sex happens between the ears." And when it does, that's mental foreplay. You'll get his imagination working long before you get to the bedroom. So what kind of sexy mind games turn men on?

* "Suggestive conversation." —Oliver, 42, educator

* "When the woman tells me that she wants to take the

initiative." —Bruce, 31, financial planner

* "Sexy talk." —Robert, 39, attorney

* "Telling me how wet she is." —Morgan, 27, financial analyst

* "Watching pornographic films together." —Pete, 42, sales

* "When a woman is verbal and honest." —Jack, 52, graphic designer

* "Active direction to her hot buttons." —George, 48, marketing consultant

* "Public teasing that goes on for hours on both parts." —Jordan, 45, marketing professional

* "Foreplay that starts well before the bedroom—like in the car on the way back from a show, touching, petting, dirty talk."
—Bob, 28, engineer

Sometimes mental foreplay isn't so much verbal as visual. "The foreplay that gets me the hottest is when a woman shows herself off while walking, moving, dancing, and making eye contact," says Serge, 27.

HE SAYS

Here's an idea. Ask your guy to tell you the last thing you did that got him all hot and bothered. You may be surprised at the answer. It could be as simple as the time you wore a white T-shirt and jeans to a party. Or maybe the time he saw your thigh peeking out of a short skirt. Take careful notes, and next chance you get, try it again. See if the dough will rise a second time.

■ ■ ■ ■ ■

TIP #2: **Keep on kissing** At the risk of sounding like a broken record, we'll say it again: Learn how to be a good kisser, and you'll have learned how to be "good" at foreplay. Men love kissing, and not just on the lips. When asked what type of foreplay gets them the hottest, guy after guy cited "passionate kissing" and "slow kissing, everywhere."

"There is nothing better than passionately kissing the woman I love with a full-body embrace, with my hand wandering down to that place where her legs and butt meet," says J.B., 50. Adds Ben, 40: "I like foreplay with lots of kissing and petting, while I slowly remove her clothes and kiss every inch of her. I want to get her so worked up she begs me to take her!"

In contrast, bad or "sloppy" kissing is "death," said men like Allen, a 35-year-old film producer. Learn to pucker up!

TIP #3: **Try sexy touching— skin deep and then some** There's his mouth, there's his member—and there's a lot of real estate in between and around. Think of his entire body as one big erogenous zone. After all, our largest organ is actually our skin. Here's the kind of physical action that gets our survey respondents in the mood:

* "A good full-body massage." —Scott, 29, student

* "Biting my nipples." —Malcolm, 34, manager

* "Intermittent touch. Sometimes hard, sometimes gentle, depending on our mood. This leads to the most anticipation." —Sam, 46, business consultant

* "Teasing hip motion." —Xavier, 40, engineer

* "Lots of groping and moaning." —Walt, 27, marketing manager

* "Slow, light contact. Lips to breast or hand to thigh—even if we're still clothed."
  —Simon, 36, programmer

HE SAYS

Try this. Seductively glide a finger across the back of his neck, or pass your hand across the small of his back, then watch his reaction. Those spots are two of his most overlooked erogenous zones.

■ ■ ■ ■ ■

* "Mutual touching all over, and then more touching and caressing, especially my neck! I like a little bit of sweet torture, with a fair amount of communication (verbal or otherwise) that 'ultimate' happiness will eventually be achieved."
  —Ted, 44, logistics manager

* "Light, slow stroking." —George, 50, attorney

* "Touching (anywhere) with a smile." —Alex, 32, manager

* "Sucking ears, nipples, stroking hair, squeezing buttocks, obviously the more 'private parts,' inside leg." —Chris, 34, software engineer

* "I love to cuddle, speaking softly to each other while our hands gently explore each other's bodies." —J.B., 50, software engineer

Note that sexy touching should be, well, *sexy*. It shouldn't hurt (unless you're into that). "For me, pinching hard or playing with previously forbidden areas takes my focus completely off sensuality," says Jordan, 45. "And when I lose focus, I lose interest."

TIP #4: **Men equate foreplay with oral sex**

When some men hear the word foreplay, they think oral sex—giving *and* receiving. (At least one of your coauthors reminds you that oral sex can be much more than foreplay. It can be an end in and of itself, especially if it leads to the recipient's climaxing!) Take a look at the way some of them answered when we asked them what type of foreplay gets them the randiest:

* "69. Plain and simple, there is nothing more sexual."
  —William, 39, business development

* "Oral stimulation on her—as long as she's enjoying it, of course—gets me as hot as her doing it to me."
  —T.J., 42, musician

* "Giving her oral sex." —Robb, 59, scientist

* "Tongue—everywhere." —P.B., 51, corporate headhunter

* "Giving oral sex!!!" —Ned, 48, retired attorney

* "Blow job." —Greg, 35, engineer

* "Oral teasing." —Allen, 35, film producer

We'll get to mouth work specifics in the next chapter. Just be aware that many guys consider oral action a great prelude to the main event.

TIP #5: **Some men aren't picky**

And then there are the men who aren't picky when it comes to foreplay. These guys aren't fixated on a particular technique (unless it's "all of the above"). When we asked them what type of foreplay gets them the hottest, here's how they responded:

* "Any." —Brian, 37, entrepreneur

* "It's hard to choose a favorite. Variety is always good."
—Mike, 23, restaurant worker/student

HE SAYS

Yes, this is true. And too often, we just dive right in, which we know is bad, but in our haste to get to the real action, we may rush things a little up front.

■ ■ ■ ■ ■

* "Watching porno. Long teases. Her dancing for me. Kisses." —Rob, 45, self-employed consultant

* "I enjoy bringing a woman pleasure and that gets me hot." —Pete, 51, artist

* "Hands on my body, rubbing through clothing, genital kissing, sexy conversation." —Marcus, 47, general manager

* "Letting me remove her clothes, engaging in a bit of sexy wrestling." —Boris, 43, creative director

* "Anything that makes her sigh or express a state of ecstasy." —Richard, 35, teacher

In fact, any kind of strenuous physical activity can be a prelude to sex. One man even cited fencing as his favorite foreplay activity. "It gets us both very turned on, as does, in general, any kind of playful romping and wrestling that turns into hot kissing," says Patrick, 40, a writer. Rugby, anyone?

Foreplay Moves to Avoid

If you're trying to get your man in the mood, what should you *not* do? Here's the advice we got from our respondents.

 TIP #1: **Drop the bad attitude**

Think an aloof, haughty demeanor fascinates men?

It doesn't. A negative attitude is a surefire way to cool his jets, no matter how hot you might look in that sexy little outfit.

"Within reason, there's nothing physical that turns me off," says Simon, 36. "But attitude can be a killer—like if she's moody or upset (not necessarily with me) or just really not into it tonight."

Treating others badly also rates high on the "turn-offs" list: "I hate when women are rude or bitchy to other people because they think it gets them more attention," says Brian, a 29-year-old filmmaker. So be nice to that waiter!

Other sexual deal-breakers:

* "When she doesn't know how to respond to sexual banter." —William, 39, business development professional

* "Giving me the silent treatment." —Kelly, 27, graduate student

* "When she applies and reapplies makeup, is extremely annoying

  (although that's hard to qualify outside of specific situations), or plays games (i.e., running hot-and-cold, or being easily and suddenly offended by certain things as opposed to just saying 'no')." —Nigel, 31, scientist

* "Boredom, even if feigned." —Gene, 64, writer

* "Smoking, checking cell phone, etc." —Ted, 44, logistics manager

* "Ongoing conflict or contention." —Dave, 41, executive

* "Bad attitude, as in bitchiness or being overly demanding." —George, 50, attorney

At the risk of stating the obvious, note that having a good attitude is especially important once you've actually reached the bedroom. No one enjoys a disinterested lover. "I don't like being rushed in bed or being given the sense that she considers sex obligatory," says Robert, 39, an attorney. Adds Philip, a 45-year-old consultant, "It definitely turns me off if she's not 'into' it."

So if you're just not in the mood tonight, be honest about it (and let him know it's not him). Chances are he'll notice if you're just going through the motions, and it will dampen his ardor, too.

TIP #2: Clean up your act

Several men named bad hygiene as their top turn-off. They love a woman's natural scent— but a clean, I-take-regular-showers kind of scent, not one that screams, "I just spent three weeks hiking through the backwoods." Patrick, a 41-year-old

HE SAYS

Guys love to look at Victoria's Secret supermodels, but most of us don't want to date them. Remember the old joke: "For every model out there, there's some guy sick of putting up with her shit." Same idea. There is nothing sexier than the right attitude. So drop the pretentious bitch act and let your hair down. I promise you'll have a great time.

■ ■ ■ ■ ■

HE SAYS

No need for a French shower,
but this is a topic that cuts
both ways, so my advice is
just to be honest. Some of us
love the musk of a woman,
while others feel it's a bit too
much. I'm sure you feel the
same about us.

■ ■ ■ ■ ■

marketing professional, elaborated: "I love going down on a woman. But if she mentions right before we enter the bedroom that she hasn't showered today, that can be a turn-off."

This doesn't mean you need to smell like the cosmetics counter at Macy's. One guy expressed dismay with women who douse themselves with "too many products—heavy perfume, heavy hair spray, too much makeup, too many chemical/floral/artificial smells (and feelings)."

You might want to steer clear of a garlic-laden dinner, too. But if you indulge, be sure you've brushed your teeth—several guys mentioned bad breath as a definite turn-off. And reconsider your smoking habit, as many men said they considered kissing an ashtray less than attractive.

A few guys even cited discussion of "bathroom issues" as a turn-off, so table the chat about your bladder and scatological habits until you've gotten to know each other a little better. (Disclaimer: Cynthia realized that she really cared about Nima when, early in their relationship, he was rushed to the ER for an intestinal obstruction. But bonding over a discussion of lower GI tract issues at your beloved's hospital bedside is a bit different from announcing on a first date that you just took the world's biggest dump.)

 TIP #3: Tone it down Here's where it gets a little confusing. Yes, men love it when you take the initiative. What they *don't* love is when you attack them like a drunken sailor on shore leave after six months at sea. Men cited aggression—"overt, tacky" aggression—again and again as the trait that would send them running for the door. "I'm turned off by a woman who's too forward and too drunk," says Scott.

"Moves like grabbing my crotch or trying to jam a tongue down my throat don't work for me," says Marcus, 47, a general manager. Pete, a 51-year-old artist, comments, "While I like a woman with healthy, open sexuality, being too loose is a turn-off."

If you're getting the sense that there is a fine line between "passionate" and "aggressive," well, maybe there is. This is when you'll just need to be sensitive to your intended lover's body language and responsiveness.

 TIP #4: On the other hand, there's such a thing as too modest The men who answered our survey crave a lover who's open, enthusiastic, creative, and comfortable with her body. Self-consciousness and prudery are surefire libido-slayers, they said. "It really kills the mood when a woman puts clothes back on *during* sex because she's 'modest' or whatever you call it," says Mike, a 23-year-old restaurant worker and student.

"Sex should be impulsive and unrestrained," comments Boris, 43. "I get turned off when she's too tidy, too preening, or too fussy about undressing and making up the bed."

"My turn-off is women who only feel comfortable in the bedroom," says Ben, 40, an architect. "What's wrong with the couch, on top of the kitchen table, in the shower, outside where you might get caught?"

 TIP #5: Avoid distracting conversation It's not just how you use your mouth that makes you a good lover—it's what comes out of it as well, according to our survey respondents. First of all, keep the complaints and

Ix-nay talking about the ex-oyfriend-bay as well. All comparisons or mentions of ex-lovers are strictly *verboten* during sex, as are topics including but not limited to: the children, household chores we promised to take care of but still haven't, why you think his mom hates you, why you don't approve of your best friend's new boyfriend.

■ ■ ■ ■ ■

negativity to a minimum. "I get turned off if she keeps bringing up concerns about her job or her living situation or things that aren't leading to seduction/love/sex," says T.J., a 42-year-old musician.

Talking about something "stressful" or "divisive" can also kill the mood, say men like Alex, a 32-year-old manager. In other words, despite what you may have heard about the joys of post-fight make-up sex, several men cited conflict as dampening their ardor.

Consider self-deprecating remarks *verboten* as well if you're trying to get romantic. "This isn't the time to get shy or suddenly tell us the ways you feel fat or ugly," advises 40-year-old Patrick, a writer.

Other conversational gambits you may want to avoid:

* "Talk about what's going to happen the next day." —Ted, 27, production assistant

* "Corny lines." —Morgan, 27, financial analyst

* "Talking about her other sexual experiences." —Rob, 45, self-employed consultant

* "Distractions, breaking up the mood by going to wash, etc." —Joe, 59, consultant

* "On a first encounter, the word *fuck*." —Serge, 27, student

* "Talking dirty. Except as a spontaneous utterance near orgasm, talking dirty always feels too contrived to me." — Ned, 48, retired attorney

 TIP #6: There's nothing you could do And then there are the guys for whom nothing is off-limits. "If I'm turned on, nothing can turn me off!" exclaims Paul, 29, a graduate student. These guys are probably the exception, but they're out there.

The Art of Kissing

If you've learned anything from this chapter, we hope it's that good kissers win at foreplay. What type of kiss gets a man really hot and bothered? Well, our survey indicates that when it comes to kissing, variety really *is* the spice of life: Nearly half the respondents to our survey said all kinds of kisses are turn-ons, whether they're deep and lingering or sweetly gentle.

Several men elaborated on their preferred kissing techniques. "I like confident kisses that are not too wet and feature some tongue and good pressure," says Andy, a 45-year-old electrician. Advises Boris, 43: "Build up from short and sweet to all of the above." Jordan, 45, likes kisses that are "light and teasing at first, but then become deep and lingering."

And then there are the guys who see kissing as a team sport. "What kind of kiss do I like? The kind that turns *her* on," exclaims Dave, a 41-year-old executive. We say amen to that!

What type of kiss do you like best?

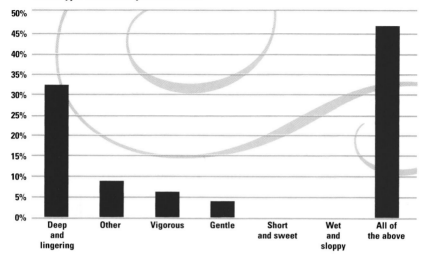

Deep and lingering	~32%
Other	~9%
Vigorous	~6%
Gentle	~4%
Short and sweet	
Wet and sloppy	
All of the above	~46%

His Erogenous Zones

While his clothes are still on (or more or less on), where should you focus your foreplay efforts? The guys we surveyed named the mouth and neck (particularly the nape of the neck) as their hottest nongenital erogenous zones. Could it have something to do with their love of kissing? We think so. Next on the list were inner thighs and ears.

Oh, and think that your breasts are fun to play with? Several men said that they'd like you to learn how to play with *their* nipples! Caution: We'd suggest checking in with your partner before you start nuzzling his nubs, because nipple play isn't for everyone. As Ned, a 48-year-old retired attorney, said, "I can't remember the source, but the line is something like 'Licking my nipples does nothing for me. A woman might as well be licking my wallet.' That's exactly how I feel. To me, the brain is the hottest erogenous zone."

What's your hottest NON-GENITAL erogenous zone?

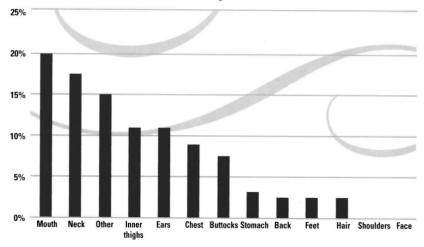

When your clothes finally do come off and you're exploring his nether regions, don't forget about the family jewels. "My hottest erogenous zone is my scrotum! It's misunderstood!" exclaims Claude, a 34-year-old musician.

When He Glimpses Heaven, What Does He Like to See?

Okay, so it doesn't really have much to do with foreplay—directly—but bikini-line grooming is such a hot topic of conversation among the women we know that we had to ask men what *they* like to see when they get your pants off. And well, girls—you'd better suck it up and embrace waxing, because 50 percent who answered like either a "landing strip"–style design or a Brazilian (the kind where everything has to go). But nearly as many guys like a standard bikini line; as long as you're well-groomed, these guys don't care how much waxing you do down there.

What kind of bikini line grooming do you prefer on a woman?

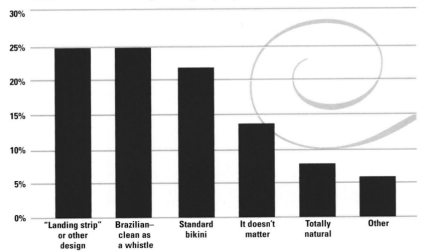

Don't think you have to find one style and stick to it. "I'm always hoping for continuous variety," says Oliver, a 42-year-old educator.

"Surprises are nice," agrees Dan, 38, a real estate agent. "I like 'all of the above' at different times."

HE SAYS

Waxing or shaving is always a fun (albeit itchy) experiment. Try a Brazilian, and if your guy likes it enough, see if he'll reciprocate. It's only fair. Shaved balls, anyone?

■ ■ ■ ■ ■

Foreplay: Anyone Can Do It

As we looked over the responses to our survey, one thing became clear: As with any shared activity—whether it's a rousing game of tennis or some serious groping on the living-room couch—when it comes to foreplay, what men want most is an enthusiastic and sensitive partner who wants to give pleasure as much as she likes receiving it. So take your time getting to the finish line!

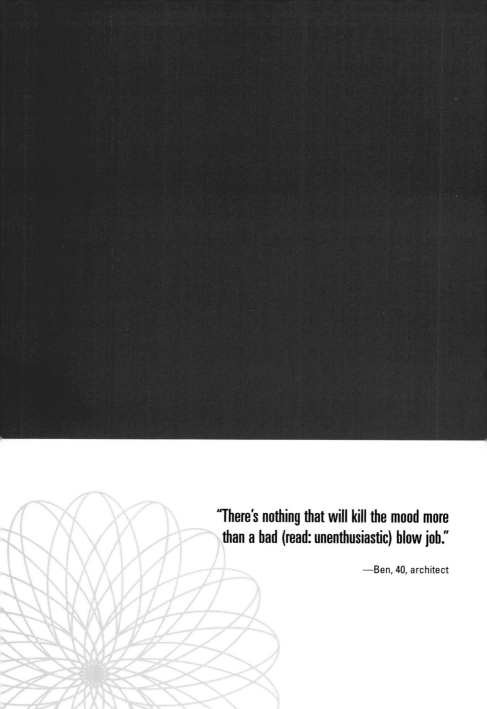

"There's nothing that will kill the mood more than a bad (read: unenthusiastic) blow job."

—Ben, 40, architect

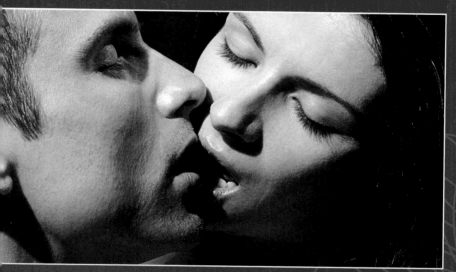

CHAPTER FOUR

Mouth Work

No surprise here: Men love oral sex—getting and giving it. "Sometimes we like it more than sex," says Alex, a 32-year-old manager. In fact, of all the men who answered our survey, only one claimed not to like it (and we're dying to ask him why he doesn't). But for the rest, "it can't happen often enough," as Rick, a 27-year-old graduate student, commented. So what are the key points men want you to know?

What Men Wish Women Knew about Oral Sex

Most women know how important oral sex is to men. And that can cause either insecurity—am I doing it right?—or overconfidence—as long as he's getting enough of *that*, I'm home free. Read on to find out the truth:

 TIP #1: **They love getting it (duh)**

One more time, with feeling: Men enjoy receiving fellatio—getting a blow job, to use the vernacular—very, very much. If you want to go down on your man, it's not likely you'll be turned down. "We love blow jobs anywhere, almost any time," says Bob, 28, an engineer.

 TIP #2: **Polish your technique (a.k.a. a little variety goes a long way)**

Having said that, it *is* possible to give a mediocre blow job. Remember that each man is different. What worked for your high school boyfriend (i.e., anything) may not work for a guy in his forties. "A woman needs to pay attention to what the man she's with likes, not just to how she knows how to do it," says Marcus, 47, a general manager. "Technique must vary by individual to get the man to respond (and come)!"

So what *is* the best technique? According to our survey respondents, it's one with variety. "There's more than one motion for cock sucking," advises Malcolm, a 34-year-old manager. "It doesn't have to just involve sword swallowing," says Jordan, 45, a marketing professional. "It's nice to mix it up." Agrees Boris, a 43-year-old creative director:

"Variety and creativity are best—there's not just one way to do it. Vary your moves and your position."

So if you really want to send him into oral heaven, mix up your rhythm, speed, and pressure. As Joe, a 59-year-old consultant, comments, "Oral sex is most erotic when done at various pressures and with suction versus motion." What guys *don't* like is inconsistent rhythm—and by that, they mean when you keep starting and stopping (no doubt because you're tired) just as they start to get close to climaxing.

There's one thing you do have to remember, though: Go deep. Don't be shy about taking his whole member in your mouth, and "focus on the shaft, not just the head," according to Ralph, a 34-year-old project manager. As Oliver, a 42-year-old educator, says bluntly, "It's not a hand job with the tip of the penis in your mouth." And while activities like licking and kissing the penis are nice extras, "most of your time should be spent sucking," counsels David, 43, a systems administrator.

That doesn't mean your focus should always be exclusively on his shaft. Some men would like you to consider the whole region fair game. According to Ned, a 48-year-old retired attorney, "It's not just about using your mouth on the head and upper shaft. It's a mix of stimulating everything from butt to tip with your mouth, hand, and teeth (lightly, thank you very much)—and using a

HE SAYS

Rent a porno. Watch it together. Ask him which style he likes, then experiment on him. Eventually, you'll be able to adapt to his physiology and blow his mind away, no pun intended.

■ ■ ■ ■ ■

What's the biggest mistake women make when performing oral sex?

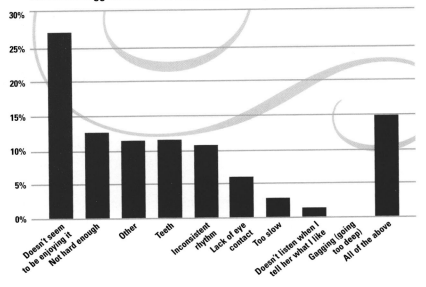

lot of spit." Adds filmmaker Brian, 29, "It's not all about sucking the shaft. There are plenty of other things to do down there."

TIP #3: **Show him that you're enjoying yourself**

In case you're worried that your oral technique leaves something to be desired, we'll put your mind at ease: All the fancy tricks in the world won't do a thing for him if you look like you're doing them grudgingly. According to the guys in our survey, the biggest mistake you can make—by far—when you're performing oral sex is to look like you're not enjoying yourself. A lackadaisical attitude is a much bigger mistake than blow-job no-nos like not applying enough pressure, inconsistent rhythm, or the feeling of teeth. "Just because you're there doesn't mean it's working," says Greg, a 35-year-old software engineer. "Put in some effort."

In fact, for most of our respondents, enthusiasm is the best "technique" you could ever master. "Enjoy it, relish it, languish in it, be creative, make it an art form," advises J.B., 50, a software engineer. "Show me that you love doing it and that there's nothing else you'd rather be doing," says Serge, a 27-year-old student.

And the more enthusiastically you approach your man's member, the better. "Play with it, slide up and down, pull back and admire it with a sexy/hungry/evil grin and do some serious licking as well as good ol' hard-core deep-throating," says Ted, a 44-year-old logistics manager.

This effort will pay off, because even though you're the one giving the blow job, your pleasure affects his. Robert, a 39-year-old attorney, speaks for pretty much everyone when he says, "If you don't enjoy it, I don't enjoy it. Don't stare up at me constantly to see if it's working. Show that you enjoy it by being confident about it. If you're diffident or looking at me for assurance, I start to feel like it's a chore for you."

"It's easy to tell if you're into it or just doing it because you feel obligated," says Ben, a 40-year-old architect. "There's nothing that will kill the mood more than a bad (read: unenthusiastic) blow job."

So even when your mouth is otherwise occupied, look up at him with pleasure in your eyes. Make noise. Show him with your body language that you love giving him pleasure. If you do, the chances are good that he'll be glad to return the favor.

 TIP #4: Take your time Please note: Enthusiasm doesn't mean that you should rush the proceedings. Take your time. Several guys said that they wanted you to make this exquisite pleasure last. Not every man wants to rush toward climax—in fact, he might need some time to get there, just as you do. "Faster is not always better," says Dave, a 41-year-old executive. "Don't hurry," says Luke, a 32-year-old student. "Start slowly and build up."

There's a practical reason for this. If the situation were reversed, you certainly wouldn't want him diving straight for your clitoris and ignoring everything around it. For one, most of his nerve endings are located in the head of his penis, making it too sensitive for a full-on attack. (In fact, the ridge between the head and the shaft is supersensitive.) So build up his anticipation. Kiss his rod and caress it with long, slow licks. Think of it as a Popsicle, not a lollipop. If he's not erect yet, pull his penis into your mouth and gently suck until it is. As he becomes hard, increase your pace and your pressure. The longer you make it last, the better!

 TIP #5: **Use your hands**   Now, if you did want to expand your oral repertoire, there's a very simple way to do it: Learn to use your hands and mouth together. Many men in our survey said that their pleasure doubles when you use your hands in conjunction with your mouth. "Hand-stroking along with full-mouth-sucking is by far the best," raves 42-year-old T.J., a musician.

Think of your hand as an extension of your mouth. Make a ring with your index finger and thumb (like an okay sign) or with your entire hand. You can either slide your hand up along his wand with your mouth, or, as you pull your head and mouth up, slide your fingers down with a tight grip. Experiment with different motions to see what drives him wildest. For example, Claude, a 34-year-old musician, notes that "the twist of the hand at the head of the cock is simply sublime."

For more ideas, Matt, a 46-year-old political activist, suggests that you "watch a porn movie to see a woman use her hands as well as her mouth. Pressure near the top is great. From masturbating, I'm used to more rough handling than you think."

TIP #6: Don't forget the family jewels

As Cynthia suggests in her book *Mind-Blowing Orgasms Every Day*, feel free to take a break from his pole to visit the twins. "Don't forget my testicles! They want attention, too!" says Walt, a 27-year-old marketing manager. So run your tongue lightly over his testicles. Slip them one at a time into your mouth and suck gently. Or simply caress them while you pleasure him orally, timing your strokes with the rhythm of your mouth.

TIP #7: It's mouth work, not tooth work

If you remember nothing else when giving a blow job, remember to cover your teeth with your lips as much as possible. While a few random guys actually liked the feeling of your teeth, most of them, like Scott, a 29-year-old student, begged you to "make sure the teeth don't get involved."

TIP #8: Wet and wild

No matter what hand technique you use, make sure that you use lots of saliva along with it. "Make sure it's nice and wet," counsels John, a 24-year-old contractor. You want the friction to be pleasurable, not painful. "Wet and sloppy is okay—it feels good," Paul, a 29-year-old graduate student, assures us.

TIP #9: It's not the be-all

Don't get too hung up on your blow-job "technique." Yes, guys love oral sex, but "not every guy thinks it's the best thing in the world," say men like George, an attorney in his fifties.

Adds Patrick, a 41-year-old marketing professional, "It's probably the last on my list of things I like in the bedroom. But with that said, a great blow job is an incredible experience."

That's because for some men, even a great blow job is just a prelude to the main event: making love. "Oral sex usually makes me want to go straight to intercourse!" says Patrick, 40, a writer. And as Dave, a 40-year-old analyst puts it bluntly, "Sometimes I'd much rather fuck!"

Finding the Best Rhythm and Pressure

No matter what kind of exotic oral tricks you perform on your man, just remember that "at a certain point, it's all about consistent rhythm," says Jordan, a 45-year-old marketing professional. "Timing and speed matter, depth doesn't," adds 36-year-old Simon, a software programmer. And for most guys, that rhythm should be "steady and vigorous, not soft and pensive," says Rob, a 36-year-old sales rep.

Nearly half the guys in our survey prefer a combination of rhythms and pressures—they love it when they don't know what you're going to do next, as long as you build up in intensity to an earth-shattering climax. Plus, using a combination "works until you find a rhythm and pressure that really do work," says Jordan. "Then the moaning takes over. However, it would probably be smart for me to use my words to say, 'Keep doing that!'"

So don't be afraid to try different things until you hit on the right recipe for his pleasure. "It's all about experimentation," adds Mike, a 23-year-old restaurant worker and student. "There is no formula for art."

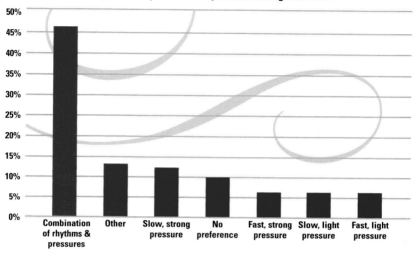

What kind of rhythm and pressure do you like during oral sex?

There's a practical reason for varying your rhythm. "Repeated sensations cause a loss of sensitivity (true of anything, actually)," claims Dan, a 38-year-old real estate agent. To some men, it also demonstrates your enthusiasm for your task. "When she varies her technique, it shows me that there's a conscious woman on the other end of the blow job, thinking about what she's doing," quips Nigel, a 31-year-old scientist.

Even those guys who checked "other" mentioned that they like a variety of speeds and pressure, although "strong pressure" was a consistent request. Of course, for some guys, it all depends on the

HE SAYS

Here's a dirty secret: Some men have "discovered" their prostates and would like you to include it in your oral repertoire. I'm not naming names.

■ ■ ■ ■ ■

situation—if you're performing oral sex as part of foreplay, you probably don't want to do something that's going to send him over the edge too soon!

How do you find out what your guy likes? "The woman needs to experiment and see how the man reacts," says Mike. "And the man needs to give vocal cues. This applies to cunnilingus, too." In fact, most of the guys with whom we spoke advised you to be observant. "Find the way to please your man by feeling his physical response and hearing his verbal response," advises 38-year-old Dan, a real estate agent. Of course, as most of our survey respondents point out, you can always *ask* your man what works for him.

Remember that your man is an individual. "I don't think there's any one thing that does it for everybody," says Patrick, a 40-year-old writer. "The best way to find out what I like is to try different things and see what I respond to, or ask me."

Top Oral Techniques

So what type of oral sex is worthy of induction into the Blow Job Hall of Fame? We asked our survey respondents to tell us about the most amazing oral technique a woman's ever used on them. Here, they describe in their own words how their woman used her mouth to take them to a pinnacle of pleasure.

She Enjoyed Herself

As several men testified, more often than not, her "technique" was simply unbridled enthusiasm for the task at hand (so to speak):

* "The most amazing oral technique? It was probably just a standard blow job. But she loved doing it and it showed. That was a huge turn-on. A *huge* turn-on! If a woman goes down on me because she feels she has to, it doesn't give me much pleasure." —Patrick, 41, marketing professional

* "The best blow job is when the woman lets herself go completely and allows herself to enjoy it." —David, 43, systems administrator

* "Focus. I just got the sense she was very happy to be down there and her attention was on what she was doing." —Matt, 46, political activist

* "She said, 'Relax, this can take as long as it needs to.'" —Gene, 64, writer

She Ordered Up the Combo Platter

Savvy women know that just because it's called oral sex, that doesn't mean you can't get other body parts (like your hands) involved:

* "She licked my nuts and used her hand to stroke me at the same time." —Bruce, 31, financial planner

* "She sucked me lightly with her entire mouth while stroking my penis with one hand and my balls with the other." —T.J., 42, musician

* "Everything. She wrapped her body around me, while kissing and sucking and caressing me with her hands at the same time." —Sam, 46, business consultant

* "She created a vacuumlike suction with her mouth and mixed it with hand action." —Joe, 59, consultant

* "She used both hands and her lips to 'pop' the head. It was unbelievable. She was practically begging me to come in her mouth, and I did." —Marcus, 47, general manager

* "She used her mouth and hand with a lot of pressure on the head and then would slide down the shaft with a consistent rhythm." —Walt, 27, marketing manager

* "She used lots of saliva mixed with her hand and mouth. It was as close to being inside a woman as is possible—in fact, it was the next best thing." —Pete, 51, artist

* "It was a combo of head-licking and slide-down-shaft-licking and then hungrily taking me while touching herself and moaning ... I think that about sums it up!" —Ted, 44, logistics manager

* "It involved tongue-circling combined with hand stroking combined with lip pressure to create a symphony of rhythm and music that forced me to lose control and not be able to anticipate what would happen next." —Dave, 41, executive

* "She slid her fingers lightly along my penis during the blow job." —George, 50, attorney

* "She coordinated her tongue and lips and hand so each maximized the effect at the right time. It can't be described in words." —Richard, 35, teacher

* "She used her hand lightly at the same time as she sucked lightly ... not to mention the fact that she looked into my eyes and made moaning noises." —Chris, 34, software engineer

* "She performed a little anal stimulation while alternating between licking and sucking my shaft and testicles." — Rob, 36, salesman

* "I like it when she licks the shaft up and down, and when she licks around the head, as well as taking as much of it as she can down her throat. I also like it when she uses her hand up and down the shaft, and cups the balls gently." —Patrick, 40, writer

She Went Deep

Work on relaxing that gag reflex, ladies. For these men, the more of their manhood you can take in your mouth (and even your throat), the happier they'll be:

* "Deep throat. The power and symbolism of seeing a woman kneel before you and take your whole cock in her mouth is off the charts." —William, 39, business development

* "I was on my back, she knelt next to me facing my feet, and it goes *way* down." —Andy, 45, electrician

* "She deep-throated me and gently tugged on me with her throat muscles." —Sam, 52, musician

* "It involved deep-throating combined with a swallowing motion in the throat." —Claude, 34, musician

* "Total deep throat." —Dave, 40, analyst

Some tips on how to perform this technique, first made famous by the 1972 Linda Lovelace movie of the same name: Widen the angle of your mouth and throat into a straight line; you may have to lie on your back with your head hanging off the edge of the bed while your man stands or kneels in front of you. You can also sit on his chest facing his feet, or assume the 69 position. The irony is that once you take his entire penis into your mouth, you won't be able to suck or lick or do much with your tongue, so deep-throating is more impressive than practical. For some guys, that's enough!

She Had Great Tongue Technique

Several men recalled how their woman's tongue dexterity sent them into paradise:

* "She used some sort of tongue-sucking method with slightly spiraling action." —Malcolm, 34, manager

* "She used her tongue from my anal region to tip of penis and back. Then she repeated it over and over." —P.B., 51, corporate headhunter

* "She slapped my penis on her tongue and left her mouth open when I came."— Serge, 27, student

* "She wrapped her tongue around me, and I honestly don't know what she did." —John, 24, contractor

Here are a few ideas (lifted from Cynthia's *Mind-Blowing Orgasms Every Day*) for tantalizing him with your tongue: Wiggle your tongue against the ridge on the underside of his shaft. Move your tongue back and forth. Dip the tip into his slit. Circle his entire member. When you reach the top of his shaft, twist your head as though you were nodding; tease your tongue against his frenulum. Suck on him as though he were a lollipop. Shake your head while sucking. Improvise, ladies!

She Had Great Rhythm
We mentioned rhythm earlier. A slow, steady pace is key to ecstasy:

* "One long dip into her mouth and one slide with her wet lips along the upper region of the organ, one long dip and one long slide, and so on!" —Clay, 31, animal control officer

* "Slow with steady pressure—she made it last a while." —Frank, 35, professional

The key is to establish a constant rhythm, gradually increasing your speed as he nears climax. Whatever you do, don't stop!

She Remembered the Family Jewels
These men fondly recalled the time their woman lavished attention on their twins:

* "She rubbed ice over my testicles during oral sex." —Chris, 45, actor

* "She swallowed my balls." —Luke, 32, student

* "Arabian Goggles (balls over the eyeballs)." —Kelly, 27, graduate student

She Knew That Sometimes, Teeth Can Be Okay
During oral sex, most men want you to keep your teeth uninvolved in the proceedings. But occasionally, a hint of

Altoids. Pop one in your mouth. Suck and chew on it for a while. That fresh minty flavor will remain and tingle and ... enough said.

your pearly whites can have an erotic effect:

* "I like feeling her teeth—pleasure and pain indivisible." —Nigel, 31, scientist

* "She used her teeth for extra friction—it felt gooood!" —Paul, 29, graduate student

She Focused on the Tip

These guys recount how women have titillated the head of their shaft:

* "She sucked the tip to make noise." —Mike, 23, restaurant worker/student

* "I don't know how exactly to describe it, but it was some technique on the tip of my penis." —Morgan, 27, financial analyst

She Gave Me Hands-Free Happiness

Yes, the guys in our survey have said, over and over, that they want you to use your hands during oral sex. But every once in a while, show him what you can do with your mouth alone. It worked for these guys:

* "She didn't use her hands at all." —Oliver, 42, educator

* "She made me come by only using her mouth, no hands involved." —Ben, 40, architect

She Liked Cold Play (and We Don't Mean the Band)
Name an oral-sex enhancer found in your kitchen. Hint: It's in the freezer. Use ice to create thrilling sensations all over his body, especially in his more erogenous zones. A few men mentioned how their woman had held an ice cube in her mouth while going down on them. Brian, a 37-year-old entrepreneur, recounted an even more exotic technique: "She hummed while holding an ice cube in her mouth. The contrast between hot and cold, and the vibrations, was incredible."

Let's put it this way—there's no end to the ways you can use your mouth to drive your man wild. Tom, a 31-year-old attorney, said that the most amazing oral sex he's ever had was when a woman "kissed and licked the head of my member after ejaculation"; for Robb, a 59-year-old scientist, the zenith of oral pleasure was simply receiving "three blow jobs in a row"!

His Geography of Desire

When it comes to mouth work, don't limit yourself to his manhood. Men enjoy the feel of your mouth and tongue all over their bodies. As we've mentioned, many men love it when you handle the family jewels—58 percent of the guys in our survey said they enjoy oral action on their testicles (only 3 percent termed the twins "off limits"). Nearly as many—54 percent—also like you to tease their nipples with your tongue. Try flicking his nipple into hardness, then blowing softly on it.

Another oral erogenous zone is the area between his scrotum and anus, known as the perineum. (Or, in the vernacular, as the taint, as in "'Taint his balls, and 'taint his

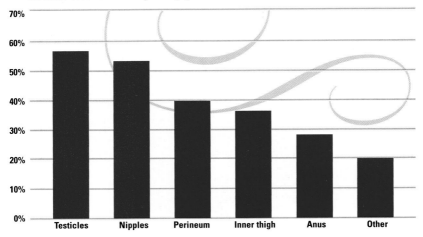

In what other areas do you enjoy oral action?

	Testicles	Nipples	Perineum	Inner thigh	Anus	Other
%	~57%	~54%	~40%	~37%	~29%	~20%

bum.") Forty percent of the guys in our survey cited this area as open for action; another 37 percent mentioned the sensitivity of their inner thighs. Several men mentioned that they like to feel your mouth on their ears and neck (Patrick, a 40-year-old writer, likes "light bites on the nape of my neck").

And for some guys, you can use your mouth just about anywhere. In fact, half of the guys who responded to our survey said that there's no area that's really off-limits for oral play. But be careful before using your tongue to burnish his bum: 42 percent said they don't want you anywhere near their anus. When you're with one of the 29 percent who do like to feel your tongue between their cheeks, make sure you're both freshly bathed and use a barrier of some sort, like a dental dam or (in a pinch) Saran Wrap.

And just how do you know which areas (other than the genitals) are primed for oral action? Just ask him, silly!

Any areas that are off limits for oral play?

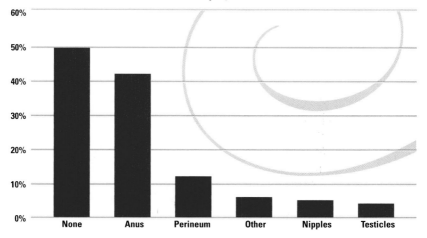

	None	Anus	Perineum	Other	Nipples	Testicles

Your other option is trial and error. Chances are good that he'll let you know if you're entering a forbidden zone. Or get playful, suggests Jordan, a 45-year-old marketing professional. "I like the game, 'Does this feel good? How about this?'" he says. "That's always been the best way for me. And, if she does it with a devilish twinkle in her eye, she's that much more likely to get a positive answer."

You could always "let him guide or coax your head to different locations," says Dan, 38, a real estate agent, but we don't think you should leave such important directions to chance.

What Men Wish Women Knew about Cunnilingus

So now you know a little bit more about how guys feel about your performing oral sex on them. (A reminder, in case you suffer from short-term memory loss: It's all good.)

Some guys think that if they take anything in the ass, it means they're gay. No. Funny thing is, they rarely have qualms about putting things in *your* ass. Help your guy embrace his prostate. Slip a finger or two in next time you go down on him, but *please* talk with him about it beforehand. You don't want a nasty surprise!

■ ■ ■ ■ ■

How do they like going down on you? Well, we can't say this strongly enough: Men *adore* lavishing your privates with oral pleasure. A full 81 percent of the guys who answered our survey say they love it, with only 18 percent claiming neutrality, saying it wasn't their favorite sex act, and a scant 1 percent saying they'd prefer not to do it at all.

"For me, it's a combination of three things," says Jordan, 45, a marketing professional. "First, hearing her moan really turns me on. Making her climax is *the* biggest turn-on. Second, the taste is usually sweet. And third, it's a 'forbidden' area of great intimacy."

How do you feel about performing oral sex (cunniligus) on a woman?

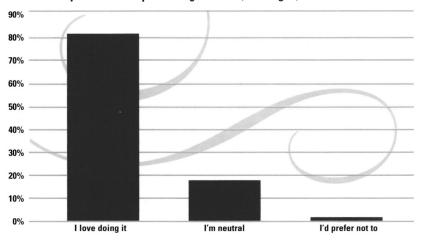

Here's what they want you to know:

 TIP #1: **He enjoys it, so relax!** First of all, if a man ventures below your belt, he's going there because he wants to. "If I say that I love it, I mean it," Malcolm, a 34-year-old manager, assures us. "I'm not saying it because I'm supposed to." Adds Robert, a 39-year-old attorney, "It's not a chore or an obligation. I enjoy it, really."

"First of all, it feels good to please somebody," says Mike, our 23-year-old restaurant worker and student. "Second, the vagina is the most intimate part of the female body. Lastly, women have their own unique tastes, and this is very endearing!"

For some guys, in fact, performing oral sex on a woman is one of their favorite sexual activities. "I really and truly do love it above almost all else," says Nigel, a 31-year-old scientist. "Long-term girlfriends finally believe me after a month or two, but often I think women have a hard time letting go and enjoying themselves because they don't really believe I like it." Gene, a 64-year-old writer, agrees: "Personally, I'd almost rather do it than almost anything else. It can take as long as it needs to, or longer."

So don't second-guess him, ladies—he's getting a lot of pleasure out of going south. "I truly enjoy doing that to a woman," says marketing exec

HE SAYS/SHE SAYS

One of my ex-girlfriends likened the art of cunnilingus to licking honey off the wings of a butterfly. That sounds pretty sappy, but I guess that's better than my previous technique, which could be likened to trying to remove a spot in the carpet with my tongue.

■ ■ ■ ■ ■

Patrick, 41. "Making her feel good orally and then sliding into her when she's all wet is my idea of a good time."

Pleasuring also plays into some men's secret desires: "Since I like being dominated, for me there's the sense that she's using me for her selfish pleasure, which I enjoy," says Nigel.

All you need to do is relax and enjoy it. "Let the man decide if you are clean enough, let the man decide when it's time to move on," says J.B., 50, a software engineer. "I think many women are hung up about cunnilingus." In fact, if you're having fun, so will he. "Enjoy it, and I'll enjoy it more," says Jordan, a 45-year-old marketing professional.

In fact, for some guys, performing oral sex on you is a prerequisite to their own enjoyment. "I have to do it to be really excited," says Dave, 41, an executive. "Her begging for it in a throaty, aroused whisper turns me on and definitely gets me into it," comments Richard, a 35-year-old teacher. And for 42-year-old T.J., a musician, "a woman's enjoyment is my biggest turn-on."

 TIP #2: Give him feedback When it comes to oral sex, how can you help your guy help you? *Tell him what you like.* Don't just lie there hoping he gets it right. We can't stress enough the importance of open communication. You don't just have to take our word for it. Listen to our survey respondents:

* "My experience is that women are all different in what they want. It's okay to tell a guy what feels good and what doesn't so that he can please you." —T.J., 42, musician

* "Tell me what works best for you. Too fast, too slow? Fingers now? Where do you want them? I'm there to make

you feel very good, and I think I do a very good job, but I need your guidance to take it to the next level." — William, 39, business development

HE SAYS

Talking is fine and dandy, but screaming *"Aaaah! Yes-just-like-that-please-don't-stop!* will generally work better.

■ ■ ■ ■ ■

* "Let me know what you like ... fast, slow, top, bottom, lips, clit sucking, etc. Some women are very sensitive, some less so, but we need to know what you like." —Marcus, 47, general manager

* "I like doing it, but I know that women are different. Let me know with words, sounds, or movements if I'm going too fast, too slow, too light, or too hard. I really want to make you have an orgasm. It makes me happy when you're happy." Matt, 46, political activist

* "I'm listening. Tell/show me what you like." —Sam, 46, business consultant

* "It's okay to tell the guy what you like and don't like when he's going down on you. Girls, most guys want to be good lovers, and if you tell them what you like, they're going to try to do it." —Patrick, 41, marketing professional

* "Speak up and let me know if something's working or not." —Allen, 35, film producer

In short, your voice is your most reliable tool for ensuring your own sexual satisfaction. Remember, your guy doesn't have ESP, and he'd love a little guidance from you.

"I have no clue what I'm doing," admits Kelly, a 27-year-old graduate student. "Give me some feedback!"

TIP #3: **Make some noise** When your man's going down on you, don't be afraid to show your appreciation of his efforts. Men find your moans of passion extremely erotic. The more you express yourself, the hotter you'll both get, as these comments show:

* "The noises she makes help me know I'm doing it right—and really turn me on." —Patrick, 40, writer

* "Don't hold back your enjoyment—talk dirty, moan, scream, play with your tits, etc." —Walt, 27, marketing manager

* "Communication is key. Let us know how close you are to orgasm, and when you orgasm, come like you mean it (make noise)." —Mike, 23, restaurant worker/student

* "You're not going to hurt my face. Move those hips!!! I love it." —Xavier, 40, engineer

There's a practical reason for vocalizing your passion. If you hold back, you could stifle the heavy breathing of your natural orgasmic response—and dampen the power of your own orgasm! So check your vocal inhibitions at the bedroom door.

TIP #4: **Practice good hygiene** Many women worry that a man won't like how they smell "down there." That's not the case—up to a point. Most guys like a woman's natural smell, but they prefer that you keep it "fresh and clean," as Rob, a 45-year-old consultant, points out. There's no need to douche: The vagina is a self-cleaning organ, and douches can disturb its natural pH balance.

"Just a quick splash of water can help," says Andy, an electrician in his forties.

But it's no big deal if you're caught off guard. "If she smells a bit 'off,' I'm not likely to stay down there very long, but I'm likely still very attracted to her and hope she won't be upset," says Ted, a 44-year-old logistics manager.

As we noted earlier, some men have definite preferences when it comes to your bikini line, as well. "Less is more as far as hair goes," says Claude, a 34-year-old musician. "I don't have anything against pubic hair in general, but it does make cunnilingus less fun," comments 36-year-old Simon, a programmer. Another musician, 52-year-old Sam, claims that shaving or waxing your pubic hair makes oral sex "the best."

But most of the guys in our survey don't care how many bikini waxes you get. "If we want to go down on you, we don't care if you just got home from work, the gym, or whatever," says Ben, 40, an architect. "We want to get you off!"

 TIP #5: Remember, he's not a robot Yes, most guys want you to relax during oral sex and not worry that you're "taking too long." Jack, a 52-year-old graphic designer, expresses the most common attitude when he assures us that "we can hang in longer than you think. It's great if you come, even if it takes a while."

On the other hand, your guy is only human. "Our jaws may get tired," says 31-year-old Tom, an attorney. Clay, 31, an animal control officer, notes that "one's neck can be put through considerable strain if one were to spend more than fifteen minutes taking care of business in the tropics." So help him out by propping up your hips, or his chest, with pillows if necessary. Suggest that he wag his head (which

Seriously girls, if it takes more than ten minutes, may I interest you in my friend BOB: Battery Operated Boyfriend. We'll even provide the batteries.

■ ■ ■ ■ ■

gives his tongue a rest while still keeping it on you) or use his finger every so often.

Be careful that you don't treat him like an inanimate object. "My head is not a bowling ball nor my ears holes for this bowling ball," says Matt, 46, a political activist. "If I'm kissing you 'down there,' please don't put your fingers in my ears!"

And know that—just as you may not have the energy to give him the world's most amazing blow job every time— he may have an off day once in a while, too. "Sometimes I'm just not into it," admits Boris, 43, a creative director. But since you're both communicating verbally about what you want, you'll know that and move on, right? Right?

And If It's All for Naught?

Even if his mouth work normally sends you over the moon, there may be times when you know you're just not going to come. Don't pressure yourself. As our survey shows, guys want you to communicate with them. Let him know how much you enjoyed yourself, and see what else is on the menu!

"First, lubrication is a good thing.
Second, you are *not* starting a lawn mower."

—Rob, 36, sales rep

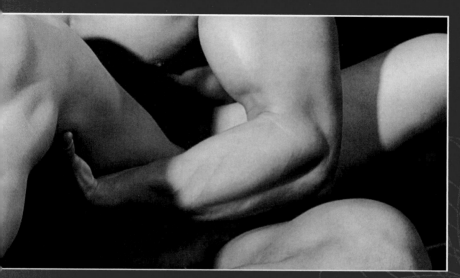

CHAPTER FIVE

▌Handy Maneuvers

You may be a pro at handling your own equipment. But how are you at handling his? Whether you're warming up to the main event in the bedroom or giving him a little surprise in a darkened movie theater, you need to know the right way to get a grip on his package. We asked men to reveal their secret longings when it comes to the fine art of hand jobs. Their candid answers may surprise you!

What Men Wish Women Knew about Hand Jobs

Once you've liberated your man's equipment from his pants, what then?

TIP #1: **Use lubricant** If you remember only one thing from this chapter, remember this: *Use some sort of lubricant.* "Grease me up!" says Rick, a 27-year-old student. It's a rare man who wants a dry rub, unless it's on a barbecued beef brisket. "Don't rub dry when there's a lot of friction," advises Sam, 52, a musician. Yes, again and again, survey respondents asserted that "lubricant is key." William, a 39-year-old business development manager, puts it succinctly: "Do *not* stroke the head and foreskin unless you have lube." Ted, a 27-year-old film production assistant, outlines the three things he wish women knew about hand jobs: "1. When to start. 2. When to stop. 3. When to use lubricant."

What type of lube should you use? It depends on what you're doing later. If you're stroking his love wand as a prelude to intercourse, use a water- and silicone-based lube (read the label). You can buy these at any pharmacy or large grocery store, or you can order them online. For the skinny on which brands are best, we went to a gay man. Our good friend Kyle Irish suggests Wet and Pjur silicone-based lubes. "They're the closest thing to oil you can get," he states.

Don't use an oil-based lubricant if you plan on having

sex with a condom, because—and this is very, very important—oil destroys latex, as Matt, a 46-year-old political
activist, points out:

"Your choice of lubrication is very important," he says.
"There are lubricants that work for hand jobs that don't
work for sex. Vaseline works for me because it lasts, but I
know I can't use it for sex because of latex condoms, so I'm
going to not want to use it unless we know that intercourse
won't be happening later. And sometimes a hand job is the
only thing that will get me off."

If, for whatever reason, you're only indulging in manual
labor, your lube options expand. You could start with hand
or body lotion, for example, although you'll need to have a
lot on hand because they absorb into the skin. "Lotion is
like training wheels," says 42-year-old Oliver, an educator.
As you get more confident and creative, you can branch
out to massage oil—or raid the kitchen for vegetable, saf-
flower, grapeseed, sunflower, or coconut oil. Our friend
Kyle says you can even use Ponds Cold Cream or mineral
oil. "You can buy them both in the grocery store, and they
feel incredible," he raves.

Of course, you can always use your own saliva
(although you must promise us to observe all safe sex
rules). This is a great choice if you're planning to embellish
your handiwork with some oral treats—but we'll get to that
in a bit.

 TIP #2: **Get a (firm) grip**   You've got your man's member in
your hand. Now what? Get a grip—a
firm one. "Don't be too gentle," advises Sam, 46, a business
consultant; think of it as a baseball bat, not Wedgwood
china. "It won't break," says 42-year-old T.J., a musician,

HE SAYS

Grab your opposing wrist
with your hand, hold tight,
and lift the entire arm.
The pressure you're
applying to your own arm is
about the most you should
use on your guy's penis.

■ ■ ■ ■ ■

"so use a fairly strong grip." Tom, a 31-year-old attorney, likens it to "gripping a golf club. Not too hard, but not too loose."

A few men in our survey offered specific pointers. "A man likes his penis enveloped, to feel its 'tube-iness,'" says David, a 43-year-old systems administrator, "so spread your fingers and grasp as much of it as you can." Fifty-year-old J.B., a software engineer, wants you to "grasp my penis firmly towards the bottom of my shaft, keeping steady pressure (but not exclusively) with your forefinger and thumb. Then stroke up and down over my head." You can either use your entire hand, with your thumb or pinkie resting against the rim, or make a ring of your thumb and index finger.

Not sure how firmly you can grip him? Ask!

 TIP #3: **But not *too* firm**   Yes, we said to get a firm grip. But there's firm—and then there's tight. Painful. "You are *not* starting a lawn mower," Rob, a 36-year-old sales rep, advises us. Adds Brian, a 29-year-old filmmaker: "It's not a stick shift. It takes some attention to detail." Dave, a 41-year-old executive, puts it bluntly: "Don't pull the knob off!"

In fact, while some men like a firm, vigorous grip, others prefer that you use a lighter touch. "Rough is not good," says George, a 50-year-old attorney. Peter, a nurse in his fifties, urges you to "be gentle and keep a rhythm." Richard, 35, a teacher, notes, "It hurts to pull the skin or squeeze too hard, so either keep it wet with saliva in generous amounts or keep your hand motion soft and gentle."

HE SAYS

Grimaces and screams of pain (from him) are good clues that you're probably holding his penis too hard.

■ ■ ■ ■ ■

Remember that it's fine (maybe even preferable) to start slow and build in intensity, as his poor staff might not be able to take an all-out assault right from the get-go. "The tip can get overstimulated," says Alex, a 32-year-old manager. So "don't go straight for the orgasm," advises Gene, a 64-year-old writer. "Light and slow for starters."

When it comes down to it, there's no need to guesstimate the amount of pressure he likes. Ask him. As Robert, a 39-year-old attorney, points out: "My penis is part of me; it's not indestructible. The idea is to stroke it where and how I tell you, not pull it off my body."

TIP #4: Different motions for different purposes

Which brings us to our next tip. The amount of pressure you use, your speed, and your rhythm will depend on your goal. Are you trying to get him warmed up for sex? Or is the hand job the main event? "Jacking me off to make me come is a different motion than when it's just foreplay," says Malcolm, a 34-year-old high-tech manager. More specifics:

* "Once we're into it, fast is good." —Nigel, 31, scientist

* "Variety is good, not just a repetitive stroke. The head is more sensitive and yields more pleasure than the shaft." –Boris, 43, creative director

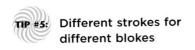

TIP #5: **Different strokes for different blokes**

Speaking of speed, the only point of agreement among our survey respondents was that when it comes to hand jobs, a constant pace—with perhaps a little more speed at the end—is the way to go. "You need to do it with a consistent rhythm," says Bruce, 31, a financial planner. "Keep the action steady: Stop-start doesn't get the job done," adds Greg, 35, an engineer.

Several men in our survey advise you not to go *too* fast (refer back to Tip #3 on page 96) until he gets close to climaxing. Then, "make eye contact and speed up," suggests Rob, a 45-year-old consultant. "Start slow and hard, and then slowly speed up until you're going fast," recommends Mike, a 23-year-old restaurant worker and student. "Slow then fast, firm pressure" is also what works for 47-year-old Marcus, a general manager.

How do you like a woman to stroke you?

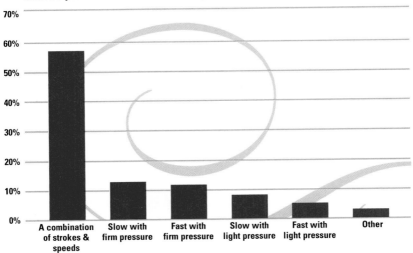

In fact, that combination of strokes and speeds is what sends the majority of men (58 percent in our survey) over the moon. "Just like with oral sex, doing the same thing over and over can desensitize me," says Dan, a 38-year-old real estate agent.

HE SAYS

You can ask your guy to masturbate for you, so you can see how he holds and strokes his little guy. After all, there's a reason Woody Allen called masturbation "sex with the person we love the most."

■ ■ ■ ■ ■

What's the best way to find out what *your* man likes? Just as with oral sex, experiment, watch his response, and if all else fails, just ask him. A little open communication never hurt anyone—especially in the bedroom.

In the end, timing is everything. "Stay attuned with how close we are to orgasm," advises Allen, a 35-year-old film producer. Gauge his responses to what you're doing. As men like Morgan, a 27-year-old financial analyst, remind us, "Don't stop too early!"

 TIP #6: Learn what he likes And because every man is so different, it pays to find out what kind of handiwork *your* man prefers. Does he want you to "touch the underside," like Robb, a 59-year-old scientist, prefers? Or would he rather you "play with the tip," like Xavier, a 40-year-old engineer, suggests? You can simply speak up: "Ask me how I like it," says Jordan, 45, a marketing professional. Or put your hand over his and ask him to demonstrate. Then imitate his moves. "You need to 'channel' a guy's hand," says Claude, a 34-year-old musician. "It can be frustrating when done too slow or too long."

HE SAYS

As with all things, practice makes perfect, so don't despair if you're not an expert at the first attempt. We appreciate the effort and love the fact that you're willing to try and learn.

■ ■ ■ ■ ■

Sometimes, you can learn what he likes just by observing. "Pay attention to the man's response," says Marcus. "The firmness of your grip and your speed need to be just right." And that's why it's so important to actually communicate (imagine!) with your lover. "Don't grab tight and yank the skin up and down!" says Ted, a 44-year-old logistics manager. "Sliding softly yet firmly without just pulling skin can be tricky. You need to talk with me and make sure we're on the same page."

Remember that as in any aspect of sex, the Golden Rule applies. "How would *you* like it to feel?" asks Pete, a 51-year-old artist. "You're imitating the act of sex, so think of your hand as a facsimile of your body."

TIP #7: It's not the be-all and end-all (most of the time)

While a great hand job can be dreamy, it's not the main attraction for many guys. "We'd rather have sex," says Dave, a 40-year-old analyst. Adds Patrick, a 40-year-old writer, "It's nice, but it will never be as good as a blow job or intercourse." Your guy has been handling his own equipment for a long time and may have specific preferences. Clay, a 31-year-old animal control officer, points out, "I can always do a better job for myself. Hell, I've been doing it since I was 13!" Some men simply prefer other ways of achieving orgasm. "A hand job should never last long," says Serge, a 27-year-old student. "That's not how I want to come."

On the other hand (no pun intended), for some guys, manual labor really works—especially when it's unexpected:

* "It's a great way to give a guy an intense orgasm. Yes, girls, we do it to ourselves all of the time, but having someone else touch us that way can feel *really* good."
  —Patrick, 41, marketing professional

* "A hand job sometimes feels better than intercourse or fellatio." —Jacques, 52, graphic designer

* "It's always better than nothing. If the woman is tired and doesn't want to give a blow job or have sex, then that will work for a guy—but be sure to use lube!" —Walt, 27, marketing manager

* "It's the surprise moment that makes it special. When you're not expecting it and it happens, it's great."
  —Bob, 28, engineer

One final note: While groping him when you're both fully dressed can be super-erotic, don't be afraid to use your hands when you're both in the buff. "It's more fun if you're naked, too," claims 23-year-old Mike.

HE SAYS

Perhaps "hand job" is a misnomer. It's really about manually manipulating your man (think about any body part that can serve this purpose other than your genitals). There's no hard-and-fast rule that it has to be just your hand and that you should only focus directly on the penis. Right hand stroking his penis, left hand on his balls, little kisses on the stomach. It's all fair game.

■ ■ ■ ■ ■

Top Hand Techniques

So what type of hand work is worthy of induction into the Hand Job Hall of Fame? Just as we did with oral sex, we asked our survey respondents to tell us about the most amazing hand technique a woman's ever used on them. Their answers fell into eight main categories:

She Did the Two-Handed Tango
While your one hand's occupied, don't sit there examining the nails on the other one. Get both your paws involved:

* "She used one hand to stroke my shaft with a slight twist at the top, while the other hand fondled my testicles."
  —Malcolm, 34, manager

* "She used both hands at the same time with totally different techniques ... It was absolutely amazing!"
  —Sam, 52, musician

* "Two hands pulling up with a twist at the end. She never pulled down. It was incredible." —Jordan, 45, marketing professional

* "Both hands in a twisting motion, well lubed."
  —John, 24, contractor

* "Oil with two hands." —Randy, 45, teacher

She Served Up a Sexual Buffet
As with oral sex, it's not an either/or equation—the most memorable hand work involved her hands *and* her mouth:

* "She stroked and sucked me at the same time."
  —Bruce, 31, financial planner

* "In combination with a blow job." Joe, 59, consultant; Peter, 58, nurse; Andy, 45, electrician; Pete, 51, artist; Chris, 34, software engineer; and many more!

* "She used lots of spit and kept her face and mouth very close." —Serge, 27, student

* "When her hand became her mouth!" —Ted, 44, logistics manager

Don't forget about the rest of the neighborhood: "The most amazing time was when she gave me a hand job while touching other parts of my body—balls, anus, etc.," says Patrick, a 41-year-old marketing professional.

She Had Mastered Her Technique

For some men, their woman's amazing technique made for a memorable manual experience:

* "She looked into my eyes while stroking me just the way I like it…. My hands were on her breasts … wow. Only one woman has ever made me come with a hand job. It was awesome." —Marcus, 47, general manager

* "The entire hand job was done while I was still wearing my underwear. She kept going for a bit after the orgasm happened. I still shudder at the thought of the pleasure of that one." —Matt, 46, political activist

* "Nothing outrageous, but sometimes she has just the right touch and timing on the underside and the head, which are so sensitive. She sort of swoops up from underneath and around and back down. It's hard to describe." —Simon, 36, programmer

* "She caressed me all over with mostly encircling down-strokes, like penetration." —Sam, 46, business consultant

* "She had an interesting thumb-and-forefinger grip." —Paul, 29, graduate student

* "She had a wet palm, she focused on the tip, and she used a technique like she was kneading dough." —Dave, 41, executive

She Had Rhythm

With the best hand jobs, the gal knew how to set a pace and keep it going. "She used firm pressure, starting slow and then speeding up as I started to breathe faster," says T.J., a 42-year-old musician. "She anticipated my excitement."

Location, Location, Location

For many of the men in our survey, their most memorable hand jobs took place in locations other than the bedroom:

* "She fondled me surreptitiously in public (in a theater, etc.)." —Patrick, 40, writer

* "On the Golden Gate Bridge." —Robb, 59, scientist

* "She gave me a hand job by a lake on a hot summer day. She used suntan oil and sent me to the moon." —Ben, 40, architect

* "Apart from necking while she gives a hand job, which beats everything, I'd have to say it's not technique, but location that matters most, i.e., a comfortable hand job in an unexpected place (like a darkened theater)." —Richard, 35, teacher

* "Getting a hand job while driving is pretty much the best."
—Bob, 28, engineer

She Remembered the Back Door

These women knew that sometimes the more "taboo" areas yield the most pleasure when combined with excellent hand technique:

* "She put a porno in, dressed up sexy, and used one hand, stroking with lube while her other hand was inside me, applying pressure on my prostate." —Rob, 45, self-employed consultant

* "While stroking with one hand, she played with my anus with her other." —Allen, 35, film producer

She Tried Exotica

Occasionally, an unexpected technique resulted in a hand job that etched itself into our respondents' memories:

* "She used this slip-on silicone 'cock sleeve' to give the hand job. Insane." —William, 39, business development

* "She moved with her entire body lying on the floor, with my penis in her hands." —Luke, 32, student

* "She sat on top of me naked while doing it." —Mike, 23, restaurant worker/student

* "She gave me a hand job while dominating me, telling me demeaning things, and making me suck her toes." —Nigel, 31, scientist

* "It was an Asian masseuse who just seemed to know about every single nerve and muscle in the general groin region and how to get the most out of it." —Rob, 36, sales

None of the Above

And then there are the men who are left cold by their ladies' handiwork:

* "I've never really had an exceptional one."
—Tom, 31, attorney

* "Yeah, right." —Xavier, 40, engineer

* "Nothing stands out." —George, 50, attorney

Masturbation: He Likes to Watch

Of course, the best way to learn how your man likes to be handled would be to watch him masturbate. Most guys—47 percent of our survey respondents—love it when you watch him pleasure himself and welcome the opportunity to show you their favorite techniques. But 35 percent of them said that while they don't mind your gaze, it doesn't do much for them. And 18 percent feel downright self-conscious about handling themselves in front of you.

It's a sad truth that many people have been conditioned to feel ashamed of self-pleasuring. He may be embarrassed to admit he masturbates without you, even though many happily coupled men masturbate regularly. To make your man more comfortable, we'd suggest moves like putting your hand over his and guiding it to his penis. Encourage him to masturbate to ejaculation on your stomach—many guys would love the opportunity to recreate this porn

How do you feel about watching a woman masturbate?

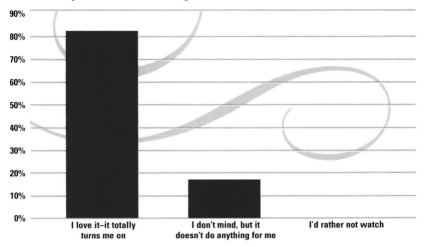

I love it—it totally turns me on	I don't mind, but it doesn't do anything for me	I'd rather not watch

movie staple. Or you could keep him company by rubbing yourself and encouraging him to do the same (a.k.a. mutual masturbation). Show your interest and excitement; reassure him that you love to watch him.

In fact, the chances are extremely good that he'd also love to watch *you* touch yourself. A whopping 82 percent of the men in our survey said that watching a woman masturbate totally turns them on. Not a single guy said they'd rather not watch you.

What is it about watching a woman touch herself that turns men on? Well, it's no more complicated than the fact that your arousal arouses him! "I love seeing a woman pleasure herself because I love seeing a woman turned on and watching her climax," says 45-year-old marketing professional Jordan. "There's also that forbidden aspect that's a bit of a turn-on, as is learning what works for her."

Comments Patrick, a 40-year-old writer, "For me, it's seeing and hearing her get aroused. I love it; I usually can't

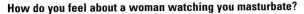

How do you feel about a woman watching you masturbate?

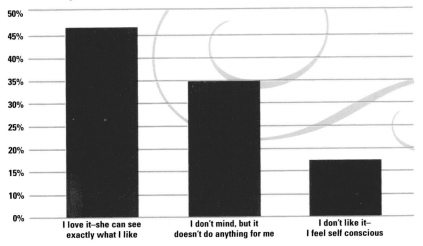

resist joining in. Sometimes I also like having her put her hand on mine and using my hand to masturbate. It's all very informative, too."

"It's a very intimate act," adds restaurant worker and student Mike, 23. "You can learn a lot. Plus, as the person watching, there's no pressure on you to 'perform' well. Then add to that all the things that make any sexual act a turn-on!"

Several men cited the learning opportunity as one of the main reasons they like to watch. "You can see her achieve ideal pleasure without it being cluttered with the idea that she has to 'share' or reciprocate," says real estate agent Dan, 38.

HE SAYS

You know how sometimes you're both a little too tired for full-blown sex, but you still need or want to come? What a wonderful occasion to engage in mutual masturbation. Less work, same results, and you still get to enjoy each other's company.

■ ■ ■ ■ ■

Let Your Fingers Do the Talking

Know that most men are visually oriented, and there's nothing more they'd like to watch than you pleasuring yourself and reveling in your sexuality. "For me, it's verification that she actually enjoys sexual activity for its own sake," says 31-year-old scientist Nigel. You'll both benefit from a hands-on demonstration. This isn't the time for shyness.

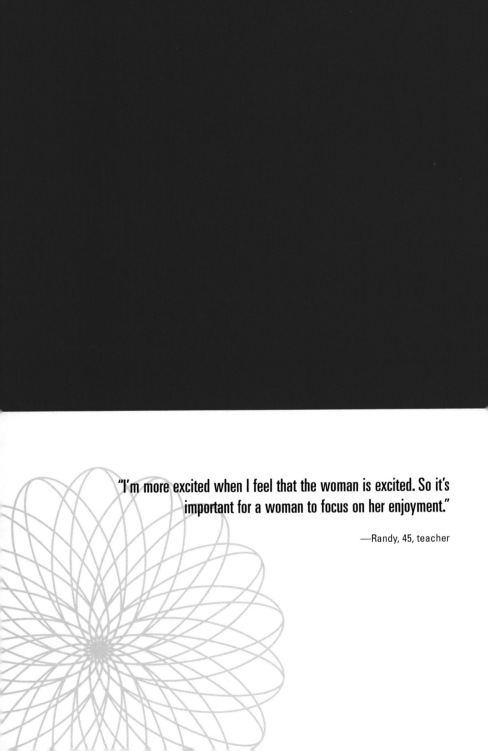

"I'm more excited when I feel that the woman is excited. So it's important for a woman to focus on her enjoyment."

—Randy, 45, teacher

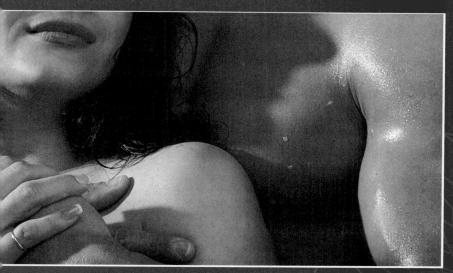

CHAPTER SIX

The Main Course

In this chapter, men dish about intercourse itself. Do they
like lots of sexy talk during the act, or none at all? What
positions are their favorites? Which would they like to try?
Do Kegel exercises really help? (If you don't know what a

Kegel is, you'll want to pay close attention.) Should you tell him if you're not getting close to the big O? We asked them these questions and more.

What Men Wish Women Knew about "The Act"

If a man had to pick the *one* thing he wished his partner knew about the act of intercourse itself, what would it be? While we received a variety of answers, one response came back loud and clear:

TIP #1: **It's more exciting if *you're* excited!**

Men want a partner who's having fun in bed. It's that simple. And the guys who responded to our survey, at least, will go out of their way to make sure you do have a good time. "I guess it keeps coming back to making sure she's enjoying it," says T.J., a 42-year-old musician. "Men hate a woman who 'lets' them do her. I think men really get enjoyment out of her enjoyment." Several others agreed with T.J., adding that they actually want you to be selfish about your pleasure—for partly selfish reasons. "I'm more excited when I feel that the woman is excited," says 45-year-old Randy, a teacher. "So it's important for a woman to focus on her enjoyment."

In fact, there's no bigger turn-off than a partner who's having sex out of a sense of obligation. "Sex should be fun, not a chore or a duty," says Brian, 37, an entrepreneur. Adds Rob, 36: "It's unacceptable to just lay there." Don't think you can fool him by faking passion, either. "Your partner can tell if you're not into it," advises Peter, a 58-year-old nurse.

For the men in our survey, part of enjoying yourself in bed is shedding any self-consciousness you might have. "Women need to let go of their inhibitions and just go for it," says 47-year-old Marcus, a general manager. "Don't worry about what I might think. Be a freak!" The more you can get out of your own head and stay in the present, the better. "Sex is a conversation between two bodies and there should be *no* thinking at all," says Andy, 45, an electrician. Sex isn't the time to worry whether you have a hair out of place: "The dirtier and sweatier the better," advises Rick, a 27-year-old student.

HE SAYS

Sex and pizza: They both taste good when cold, but they're so much better when *hot*.

■ ■ ■ ■ ■

Yes, sheer enthusiasm wins out over any fancy technique. "The one thing women should know is how friggin' incredible sex feels to a guy," says Patrick, a 41-year-old marketing professional. "And there's no 'bad' position as long as both people are into it."

TIP #2: **They want you to come, really**

Guys don't want you to just enjoy yourself in bed with them. They want you to *really* enjoy yourself by having a mind-blowing, rip-roaring climax. Repeat after us: It is *not* selfish to focus on your own orgasm. "Women should prioritize their orgasm, because a guy is going to have one no matter what," says Walt, 27, a marketing manager. "And it's a huge turn-on to hear a woman come." Jordan, a 45-year-old marketing professional, agrees. "Don't hold back," he says. "Let's see how many times you can climax. I can only climax once, so let go and enjoy it. The sexiest thing you can say is 'I'm coming!'"

TIP #3: It means something to them

Despite what we hear and see in the media about men and sex, "men aren't in it just to get off!" say guys like Sam, a 52-year-old musician. Jack, a graphic designer also in his fifties, concurs. "We're interested in more than that—really," he says. Steve, a 27-year-old student, adds, "There's more going on than just intercourse." At the same time, men like Pete, a 42-year-old sales rep, remind us that sex "is not always a commitment."

TIP #4: Variety is the spice of life

If you've got a good thing going with your mate, it pays to mix things up every once in a while. A common refrain among the guys who responded to our survey was that variety is key to keeping sex exciting. "Too much of one position gets old and boring," says Claude, a 34-year-old musician. So don't be afraid to roll him over every once in a while. "It's fun to go through several different positions before I'm done," comments 40-year-old Patrick, a writer.

At the same time, don't pressure yourself to write sexual history every time you make love. "Every time should not be an athletic pinnacle of romantic bliss outdoing all previous acts of sex in the history of the universe," says Robert, a 39-year-old attorney. "Sometimes it's fun just to have sex."

HE SAYS

If guys just wanted to "come," then we'd stay on the couch watching our porn while stroking our Johnsons. Yet we go through all the effort of cleaning up, taking you out to fancy dinners/clubs/parties, and feigning interest in all your issues and irrational fears because when it comes down to it, we like sex with you so much more than sex with ourselves.

■ ■ ■ ■ ■

Communication is key

All the fancy sexual positions in the *Kama Sutra* are useless if you're not talking to your partner about what turns you

HE SAYS

Best lie a woman ever told me was "Ooooh, I've never tried *that* before!" I knew it was a lie, but it made me feel like a sexual champion.

■ ■ ■ ■ ■

on in bed. "Communication is the key," says film producer Allen, 35. The guys in our survey want you to guide them to your pleasure zones. "Be honest about what you want so he can learn what you need," advises Dave, a 41-year-old executive. Says J.B., a 50-year-old software engineer, "You don't have to fake it. I'm sure we can find a way for you to come. Help me find it."

Speaking of which, if you are getting close to climaxing—by all means, let him know! "I like a woman to talk to me a little—I want to know where she is," says Brian, a 29-year-old filmmaker. "If she's close to coming, I want to know so I can time it and come at the same time."

In fact, by speaking up, you'll make it more likely that you *will* achieve perfect timing. Says Ted, a 44-year-old logistics manager: "Believe me, honey, I want to 'last' for you forever, and would love it if we come at the exact same time, but I'm only human (male!) and might lose control if we don't talk and keep each other 'informed.'" Most men would like it to last longer, says Simon, a 36-year-old programmer, "but our reflexes are such that it takes extra communication for this to happen." Let him know, too, whether you're up for a quickie or an extra-long session. "Give us some clue how long you'd like lovemaking to last," requests Richard, a 35-year-old teacher, "and then cooperate with us to make that happen, since different techniques will affect whether we reach a quick finish or go long."

Remember that you're human, too. It's okay to alert him to the fact that you're running out of steam as well (in a nice way, of course). "By all means, let us know when you've had enough!" says David, 43, a systems administrator. Alex, a 32-year-old manager, concurs. "Give us warning before you get tired or sore," he says.

Last but not least, don't forget that communication isn't just about giving directions—it's also about communicating how much you're enjoying yourself. "Let loose, act like a slut, scream, talk dirty, be real into it," Rob, a 45-year-old consultant, encourages women. "Noise is good," says Mike, a 23-year-old restaurant worker and student. "Feel free to scream out."

 TIP #6: Take some initiative! Although we've covered this elsewhere, it's worth saying again: The majority of men want you to make the first move every once in a while. "It's really hot when the woman takes the initiative," says Chris, a 34-year-old software engineer. "I wish women knew when to take charge (or that they can take charge more often)," adds Ted, a 27-year-old production assistant.

HE SAYS

Verbose feedback is nice, but not always necessary. On the other hand, just lying there and whimpering is bad. It makes us think we did something wrong.

■ ■ ■ ■ ■

Think how exhausting it would be if you always had to make the first move or think of new ways to spice things up. "We're always looking to try new things," says Paul, a 29-year-old graduate student. "Take the initiative. It's almost guaranteed we'll love whatever you suggest." As Boris, a 43-year-old creative director, points out, "Experimentation is fun. Try different positions, and share in taking the initiative."

Taking control may also ensure that you get more of what *you* want in bed, and it's unlikely that your man, if he has any sensitivity at all, will object to your furthering your own pleasure. "I like when a woman controls the speed," says Matt, a 46-year-old political activist. "I'm very sensitive to her needs, and if she is in control, I know I'm not going too fast or too hard and that she's lubricated enough."

TIP #7: Pace yourself Keep in mind that when it comes to sex, timing is important. If you want a long, tender lovemaking session, start out slow. "If we gear up slowly, I can last as long as you want," says William, a 39-year-old business development manager. "If you want to be pounded hard and fast from the get-go, then it's going to be a much shorter event." After all, as Gene, a 64-year-old writer, reminds us, "There's no rush." Remember that your partner is a human, not a machine. "I just can't do it for hours and hours," says Robb, 59, a scientist.

TIP #8: Do it a lot! If you want to increase the chances that your guy will last, increase the frequency of your lovemaking sessions. A guy who's starved for booty (what's known as "pent-up demand" in business terms) won't be able to last as long as one who gets some on a regular basis, according to some of the men in our survey. "If you don't do it often enough, the time it takes for the guy to ejaculate gets shorter as time goes by," claims Clay, a 31-year-old animal control officer. "Hence for maximizing their pleasure, she needs to engage more often than not!"

HE SAYS

Hah! Not even Sting can go for hours on end. He recently admitted that his last eight-hour Tantric lovemaking session was actually dinner and a movie, the drive back home, four hours of begging, and then sex.

■ ■ ■ ■ ■

As P.B., a 51-year-old corporate headhunter, puts it succinctly: When it comes to sex, "more is better."

 TIP #9: **Different guys like different things**

Many of the comments we received couldn't be grouped into any of these categories. So for what it's worth, here are some more points men want you to know about intercourse:

* "Intercourse is just one part of the entire seduction. Switch between intercourse and oral, work on other senses, like touch, hot/cold, taste, etc." —Bob, 28, engineer

* "Intercourse is best in the afternoon, when you're rested but not too sleepy, sober, present, and there's a nice natural light for exploring." —Ned, 48, retired attorney

* "It's a visual thing for a guy—I can't always do it in the dark." —Oliver, 42, educator

* "Some of the best sex is when you're on your period. The women I've done this with said that the sex is amazing." —Ben, 40, architect

* "That pelvis contact is about the most important thing for a woman's satisfaction ... that grinding is the real deal ... not just pumping and pumping. No. Wait. I guess that is what a man needs to know." —Pete, 51, artist

* "Lubrication is good for both of us." —Malcolm, 34, manager

Favorite Positions

We asked men to name their favorite position for sexual intercourse. We thought they'd name the missionary position—that is, him on top—as their number-one position. But surprisingly (or maybe not so surprisingly), they'd rather have you on top or do you from behind while you're on your hands and knees.

HE SAYS

Surprisingly, lube can also be used to slow things down a bit. If you're lubed up, there isn't as much friction on the sensitive parts, so your love-making sessions can last longer!

■ ■ ■ ■ ■

Woman on Top

Think he's threatened by your rolling him onto his back and hopping on for a ride? Think again. Thirty percent of the guys who answered our survey cited "woman on top" as their favorite position. Their reasons fell into a few general categories.

What's your favorite position for sexual intercourse?

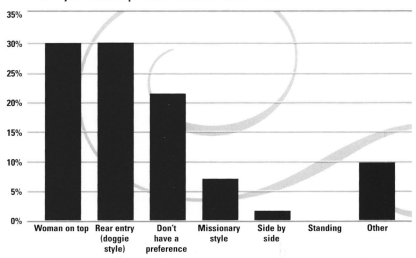

119

First of all, there's the view:

* "Great penetration. She is more active than in missionary, and I can see and touch her tits." —William, 39, business development

* "I can look at her. The sight of a naked woman sitting up above me is incredibly erotic." —T.J., 42, musician

* "1.) Stimulates her better; 2.) I can see her better; 3.) I can hold out longer; 4.) We can both move more." —Nigel, 31, scientist

* "I enjoy being able to watch her face and grab her breasts." —Scott, 29, student

* "I love watching her up there grind away on me, positioning herself how *she* likes it and getting herself off." —Paul, 29, graduate student

* "I like the view of a woman's face and body in that position, and I can reach with my hand and mouth all the parts I like, from hair and mouth to breasts, belly, or hips." —Richard, 35, teacher

  Guys also realize—and like—how much pleasure this position gives *you*:

* "Women typically have more success with orgasms on top, which takes a lot of emotional pressure off me. She's in control." —Robert, 39, attorney

* "Body contact, eye contact, breast contact, best penetration and control for the woman." —Sam, 52, musician

* "My girlfriend gets off on it." —Kelly, 27, graduate student

* "Because it's the easiest way for a woman to get off. Men just get off as a matter of course ... it's just a matter of time." —Pete, 51, artist

* "Probably because this allows the woman the most control over the feeling, and it's always wonderful to see a woman writhing on top of you in pleasure. Also feels great for the guy with maximum penetration." —Rob, 36, salesman

Make no mistake; It feels good to *him*, too, when you're on top. "It seems to provide the best contact and pressure for me," says Joe, a 59-year-old consultant.

Rear Entry

An equal number of guys—30 percent in our survey—love coming at you from behind. Their reasons varied, starting with the great view:

* "I love holding her hips and watching my member go in and out." —Malcolm, 34, manager

* "I love to watch her buttocks as well as my penis going in and out of her vagina." —John, 24, contractor

* "I like to see myself between her ass cheeks and have her looking back at me." —Morgan, 27, financial analyst

* "Like to see that booty." —Ron, 29, student

* "I can watch her hips move; also, it gives us more freedom for us to move around." —Simon, 36, programmer

They also cited the pleasurable sensations it gives them (and again, the great view):

* "It feels good. I can grab those hips and go!" —Xavier, 40, engineer

* "It just feels incredible, the pressure is just right, her ass is right there, and her breasts are still accessible."
  —Andy, 45, electrician

* "Physical pleasure, great view of the woman's body, and there are lots of things you can do with the position."
  —Serge, 27, student

* "It feels the best and I love being able to look at the woman's ass." —Walt, 27, marketing manager

* "It feels totally different than any other position. I like the view of the woman's butt and back. It's animalistic!"
  —Ben, 40, architect

* "It's usually the tightest." —Brian, 29, filmmaker

  For some men, rear entry gives them more control (and guess what, a great view):

* "It takes me a while to ejaculate, thus it allows for me to control the speed and pace. Furthermore, I love to grab her ass while penetrating." —Bruce, 31, financial planner

* "It feels naughtier, and I have more control." —Allen, 35, film producer

* "Power, view, and control." Dan, 38, real estate agent

  And for many guys, the sight of your buttocks is their biggest turn-on (in other words, they like the great view):

* "I'm a butt guy." Tom, 31, attorney

* "I love a woman's ass!" J.B., 50, software engineer

We went back to our friend, the brilliant anthropologist Dr. Timothy King, and asked him for his thoughts about why men seem to prefer the rear-entry and woman-on-top positions over missionary. In his view, what it comes down to is this: As a species, we're hardwired for rear entry, but as we've evolved, we've come to prefer face-to-face positions.

"Doggie-style," Dr. King says, "is the default mammal position. We're still wired for this position rather strongly— our equipment has adapted to this position over millions of years (as mammals), and so it usually feels good."

By contrast, the missionary and woman-on-top positions are newer ways of having sex. (Interestingly, chimps and bonobos, our evolutionary next of kin, also have sex this way.) The reason? "In our neck of the primate world, sex is not just for reproduction; it's also for social bonding," says Dr. King. "Some statistics indicate that only a very small percentage of human, chimp, and bonobo sexual encounters have reproductive ends." To put it bluntly, we have sex to socially bond, and humans are wired for having sex longer than any other mammal. Our bodies have even changed over time to accommodate longer and more enjoyable sex.

"Because sex is social bonding, and we humans have evolved to be really good at it," says Dr. King, "we've also taken to having sex in positions that allow 'face-to-face' visual contact, which may enhance the bonding experience by allowing us to look at each other."

Here's where scientific theory gets interesting. According to Dr. King, some researchers have proposed that human women's breasts are large (comparatively) and act as visual signals because of our shift from doing it doggie-style to having sex in other positions. "The idea is that a woman's bent-over ass is universally and innately arousing," says Dr. King. (If you don't believe him, refer back to chapter 2 on page 30, where we discovered that a majority of guys find your buttocks to be the sexiest part of your body.)

What happens if you shift away from rear-entry sex? Because face-to-face sex is important for bonding—which is why it tends to feel more "intimate" than, say, doggie-style—one proposal is that breasts have taken on the arousing shape of a woman's buttocks. (Our evolutionary next of kin, Dr. King points out, don't really have external breasts.) Another theory is that breasts have become some kind of new signal: Early on in our history, breasts were mildly arousing, but they now have become large over time to amplify their erotic signal and to be equally arousing as the buttocks, making face-to-face sex even more appealing.

If you follow this line of thinking, missionary and woman-on-top positions should be equally interesting to men. Why does our survey indicate something different? "My guess is that it comes down to cultural issues," says Dr. King. Doggie-style being on the top of the list is not surprising. "Missionary is looked upon as old and unadventurous. Perhaps woman on top has the same face-to-face dynamic, but it's more novel in modern culture. The woman-on-top position is more interesting than missionary, and it has the same visual signals (for men), but it's not the same lame sex that your parents were having. That's my long-ass guess." No pun intended.

No Preference
(It's All Good)

Of course, for some guys, any position is a good position, as 21 percent of the men in our survey indicated:

* "I like all the positions that let me get really deep—her legs on my shoulders, her knees together and feet on my stomach, doggie-style, one leg up and one down, etc."
  —Patrick, 40, writer

* "I like surprise and variety." —Sam, 46, business consultant

HE SAYS

I feel compelled to plug the "77," a sexual position Cynthia invented that was featured on the cover of the November 2005 issue of *Cosmopolitan* magazine. Basically, it's "spooning," but a lot less innocent. You lie on your sides, your guy behind you. Then you wrap your top leg around his and pull him close as he enters you and the two of you bend together at the waist, changing the angle of penetration so that his member hits your G-spot. Now you see why I'm the envy of my friends, who are still under the impression that life at our house is one long sexual marathon.

■ ■ ■ ■ ■

* "No preference, depends on the woman and how our bodies work together." —David, 43, systems administrator

* "I didn't pick one. It all depends on context." —Gene, 64, writer

* "They're all good." —Jacques, 52, graphic designer

* "It varies; sometimes one feels better than another." —Jordan, 45, marketing professional

* "I like them all and just change up which ones I do when." —Bob, 28, engineer

Missionary Style
Yet only 7 percent of the men who answered our survey said that missionary was their favorite position, mostly for the control it offers:

* "Because we can also touch each other on the chests." —Luke, 32, student

* "It offers better control." —Robb, 59, scientist

* "I can get in very deep and strong and as hard as I want! I'm in control and I like it that way." —Marcus, 47, general manager

* "It's the best-feeling position." —Alex, 32, manager

Side by Side
A few men enjoy lying beside you during lovemaking (think about spooning). "It allows me to use my hands, and it's slow and comfy," says Chris, a 34-year-old software engineer.

Other Positions
Ten percent of the men who answered our survey couldn't pick a single position, or listed alternative positions as their favorite:

* "Missionary is number one because it feels the best to me physically and it's the most intimate. Doggie is nice because it feels good and it can have a 'naughty' feel to it. And the view is incredible. Side by side is a great way to start off the morning; it can be tender; and you can rub

things with your hands." —Patrick, 41, marketing professional

* "The woman's preference is more important. The more her enjoyment and excitement, the more mine." —Randy, 45, teacher

* "Woman on bottom, but with her legs up alongside my head. You can go really deep, and you can see her buttocks, too."
—Mike, 23, restaurant worker/student

* "Man lying down on back, female facing the other way."
— John, 24, contractor

* "Variety is best. Repetition of the same thing is boring."
Boris, 43, creative director

* "Her on side, me on knees. It feels the best." Greg, 35, engineer

* "I work with what she needs. If it works for her, I'll get what I need." Dave, 41, executive

What He'd Like to Try

When it comes to the positions he'd like to try, the answers were all over the map—and a number of men claimed they couldn't think of one because they'd "tried them all." In fact, our survey respondents appear to be an experimental and open-minded group, with several men echoing the sentiments of 23-year-old Mike, a restaurant worker and student: "I honestly can't think of one I haven't tried. If the woman has any ideas, I'll try it." Added Marcus, a 47-year-old general manager, "I feel like I've tried them all ... sitting, standing, reverse cowgirl, side, you name it! When I look at the positions in the *Kama Sutra*, there are a few that just don't look very comfortable, so I'll just pass on those."

Now that we mentioned the *Kama Sutra*, a couple of men expressed a desire to explore the positions it describes ("but I need to get more flexible first," says Jordan, a 45-year-old marketing professional)—so girls, pick up a copy today!

Several men mentioned they'd like to try anal sex—with at least one man confessing to a fantasy where he was on the receiving end of his girlfriend's strap-on dildo.

More than a few guys said they'd like to try standing positions. "I've done it and love it," says Ted, 27, a production assistant. Patrick, a 40-year-old writer, said that sex while standing is one of the few positions he hasn't experienced. "I'm lucky in that we've tried a lot of fun positions," he says.

Some of our respondents expressed a desire to make better use of the furniture. T.J., a 42-year-old musician, said he'd like to try "me sitting in a chair with her straddling me," while Kelly, a 27-year-old graduate student, said he'd like to try "her on top facing outward while I'm sitting on a chair."

Some men also mentioned variations on common positions: "I'd like to try rear entry against a wall mirror, so I can reach around to gently fondle her breasts or finger her clitoris, touch and admire her beautiful feminine back, and at the same time still get to look into her eyes and see all the other parts I like," says Richard, 35, a teacher.

And of course, no survey would be complete without a few zany responses (depending on your point of view): Men mentioned wanting to try positions like "aerial doggie," "floating in zero-gravity," "standing in a hammock," "wheelbarrow style," "upside down," and "hanging swing and ergonomic chairs." One man described wanting to try a position that would feature "the woman on her head with back propped up against couch, legs folded over with feet on either side of head." (He doesn't say whether her feet would be on either side of his head, or her own.)

It's All about Location

Where do men like to have sex? Hands down, they prefer the bedroom: 52 percent of the guys in our survey picked it as their favorite location for making love. They cited comfort, familiarity, and convenience as the main reasons: "You can change positions easily, and your knees don't hurt," says T.J., a 42-year-old musician. Adds Randy, a 45-year-old teacher, "It's soft, intimate, and familiar." To some men, the bedroom is the most romantic spot in the house: "Other locations can be hot and erotic, but the bedroom is best for making love," says Jordan, 45, a marketing professional. This is a sentiment that J.B., a 50-year-old software engineer, expands upon when he says that "there's nothing like making love to the woman you love in your own bed." In fact, sex in public places fails to thrill many of our respondents. "The excitement of getting caught is more like a source of anxiety for me," says Robert, 39, an attorney.

And with experience and maturity also comes an appreciation for creature comforts: Sam, a 46-year-old business

What's your favorite location for sex?

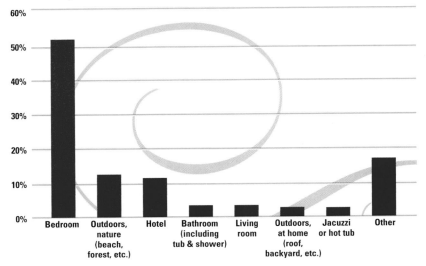

consultant, says that he prefers the bedroom because "I'm a grown-up now, and I'm delighted I don't have to resort to cars, hotel rooms, and so on, to find some private space." William, a 39-year-old business development manager, pointed out the erotic possibilities: "If you've created the right bedroom, it is the most sensual place to make love. It's private, and you can make it sexy with candles, paint color, a great bed, etc."

The next most popular place for lovemaking was the Great Outdoors—12 percent of our respondents said they like getting *au naturel* at places like the beach or while camping. "Outdoors anywhere is sexy," says Dave, a 43-year-old systems administrator, while Jack, a 52-year-old graphic designer, says that "my all-time most erotic experiences have happened outdoors."

And where better to get romantic than a room whose focal point *is* the bed? That's what another 11 percent of our respondents seemed to be thinking when they chose hotels as their favorite spot for romance. "You can be as noisy and messy as you want," says 23-year-old Mike, a restaurant worker and student: "If you're on vacation, you probably don't have any time constraints. You have a bed and a shower."

If you're at home and tired of the bedroom, there's always the living room, mentioned by 3 percent of our respondents. Take advantage of its erotic possibilities; as Rob, a 45-year-old self-employed consultant, points out, "You can have candles, a fireplace, and a 57-inch TV for porno; there are many things to bend her over; and she can dance for me." Of course, there's also the possibility that you get so hot for each other that you don't make it to the bedroom: "I think it's just that we tend to be there when we

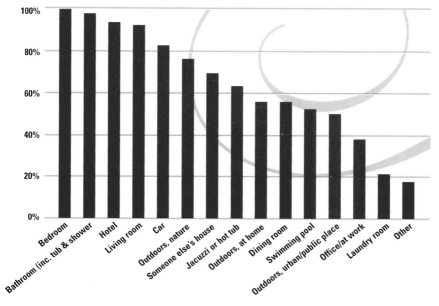

In what locations have you actually had sex?

get carried away, and so my experience of that is more exciting," says Simon, a 36-year-old programmer.

And what about the men who answered "Other" when we asked them about their favorite spot for nookie? Most of them echoed the opinion of Claude, a 34-year-old musician, who said that "anywhere is good—I'm a guy!" To these men, spontaneity is the most important element. "I don't like having sex all the time in the same place, whereas surprise and spontaneity are sexy, so I like to vary the location," says Richard, a 35-year-old teacher.

Men may have their favorite locations for sex, but where have they actually done the deed? The most common spot was—no surprise—the bedroom (every man who answered our survey has done it there), followed by the bathroom (including the tub and shower), hotel, and living room. Less popular among our respondents were public places, the office, and the laundry room (apparently the vibrations of the dryer leave men cold).

Other locations for love cited by our respondents: the kitchen, the bathroom of a nightclub, an empty classroom, a truck stop, an airplane (the famous "mile-high club"), "in a traffic jam with the convertible top down," on a pile of coats in a closet, in the rain, on a Greyhound bus, on a boat, and even—gasp—in church! (Must've been *some* sermon!)

Speak Up!

We've said it before and we'll say it again: Men *like* to hear the sounds of your pleasure. The majority of guys who responded said that they want to hear you moan and groan while you're in bed with them. They also want you to give them plenty of instruction: As long as you're not a drill sergeant about it, they *want* you to tell them what you like. "Moaning is best, but instruction is good," says 35-year-old Richard, a teacher. (Please note that not *a single man* in our survey wanted you to remain completely silent, although some found it incredibly sexy when you *try* to keep silent but can't.)

Speaking of instruction, what's the best way to show a man what you want in bed? (And they do want you to show them what you want—again, not a single man was so self-confident that he wanted you to refrain from giving him pointers.) The vast majority—70 percent—like it when you mix verbal cues ("A little to the right ... keep going ... there! Oh, God, right there!") with nonverbal cues like moaning, groaning, or however else you like to raise the rafters when what he's doing sends you over the moon.

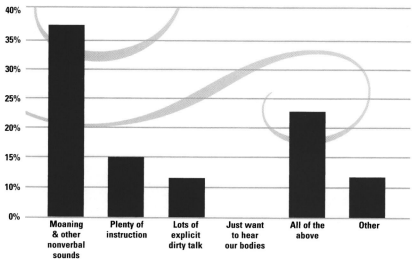

What kind of verbal action do you like during sex?

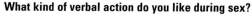

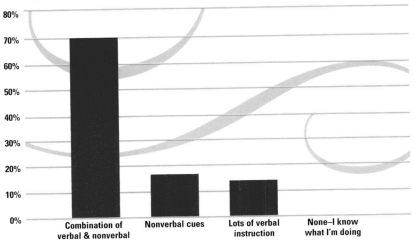

What kind of instruction do you want her to give you during sex?

80%	
70%	
60%	
50%	
40%	
30%	
20%	
10%	
0%	

Combination of verbal & nonverbal | Nonverbal cues | Lots of verbal instruction | None—I know what I'm doing

The Truth about Orgasms

Lots of—maybe most—women think they'd better pretend to be having a fabulous time, or their guy will feel like a failure and maybe blame it on them, even to the point of ending the relationship. Well, ladies, here's a piece of good news: Guys really want you to tell them if you're not getting close to having an orgasm. Of the guys we surveyed, 98 percent ask that you let them know so they can try to please you better. Isn't that a relief? Only 2 percent said it wasn't a big deal. Just remember the importance of good, considerate communication—and let him know when you're having a good time, even if it doesn't seem to be taking you all the way to the big O.

If You're Not Going to Make It, Don't Fake It

Whatever you do, don't fake it: 82 percent of the men we surveyed say it's never okay for you to fake an orgasm,

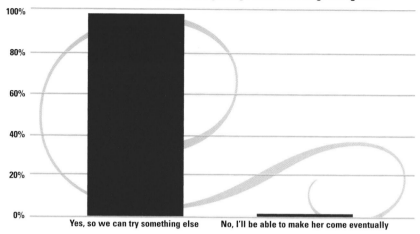

Should a woman tell you if she's not getting close to having an orgasm?

- Yes, so we can try something else
- No, I'll be able to make her come eventually

because they don't want to think you like something that you don't. And once they do, it's going to be hard for you to stop in the middle of the action and announce, "By the way, that's never really worked for me."

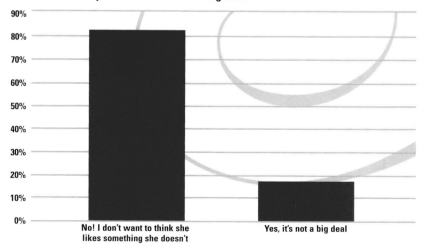

Is it ever okay if a woman fakes an orgasm?

- No! I don't want to think she likes something she doesn't
- Yes, it's not a big deal

Interestingly, however, a little more than *half* the men in our survey said that they themselves have faked an orgasm. (How is it that their partners didn't know? The mind reels.) Their reasons for doing so might sound familiar: They were tired, bored, or drunk, or they felt pressured and wanted to get it over with—without hurting their partner's feelings. Here are some of the comments we got when we asked them to elaborate:

* "I don't really 'fake' orgasms, but sometimes I know I'm just not going to ejaculate (usually because I've come too many times already or am just too tired), so I just enjoy the sensation and make my usual happy growls and leave it at that." —Patrick, 40, writer

* "My first time, it wasn't going to happen, but I didn't want to just quit." —Mike, 23, restaurant worker/student

* "Sometimes it takes a while to come, or you're not going to come because you're dehydrated or something, and she might be getting sore, and some women get 'weird' (i.e., have feelings of inferiority) when the male partner doesn't come. When you wear a condom, sometimes this is the best option. I feel I'm not hypocritical after answering that I don't think it's okay for a woman to fake an orgasm just because it happens with me so infrequently and I can't ever think of a time when I had sex and thought I wasn't sufficiently satisfied." —Nigel, 31, scientist

* "The woman was so bad at sex. I had to do all the work, and I was getting tired, so I faked it." —Bruce, 31, financial planner

* "She seemed to really want me to, but I was very tired." —
  —T.J., 42, musician

* "To get it over with when I wasn't enjoying having sex at
  the moment." —Sam, 52, musician

* "I was too tired to go on. This has happened only twice in
  my life. One was after having come twice already and,
  while I was hard, I didn't think the third time was worth
  the effort. The second was after back surgery under the
  influence of narcotics. The girl I was with wouldn't understand and I didn't want to explain." —Robert, 39, attorney

* "I was too drunk and tired to actually come; I'd been ham-
  mering away for ages and just wanted to wrap it up."
  —Paul, 29, graduate student

* "It was during marathon sex and I couldn't get one more ...
  and she really wanted to get it, and I did not want to
  explain or for her to feel bad." —Rob, 45, self-employed
  consultant

* "During phone sex, I was more interested in her getting
  off." —Ned, 48, retired attorney

* "I came too quick and tried to pass it off like I didn't."
  —Brian, 29, filmmaker

* "I thought I was going to come and I didn't—so I felt less
  stupid pretending I did." —Simon, 36, programmer

Have you ever faked an orgasm?

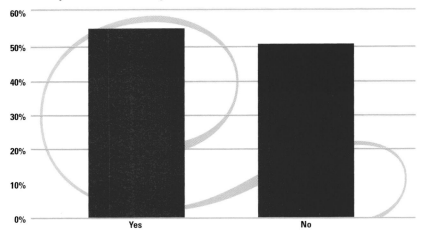

But a nearly equal number of guys don't see the point of faking it. "Why would I?" asks Clay, a 31-year-old animal control officer. "It's not like she can't figure it out." Andy, a 45-year-old electrician, asks, "You know I'm a man, right? We always get off."

What's more, many guys said that they don't enjoy sex any less if they don't climax. "I don't always need to orgasm," says Boris, a 43-year-old creative director. "If it isn't going to happen, it's fine. Sex is still enjoyable."

And many believe that honesty is the best policy—because in the long run, it results in better sex. "Honesty leads to communication and better odds for the next time," says Sam, 46, a business consultant.

Multiple Orgasms: Fact or Fiction?

When it comes to sex, there's one way in which women are very, very lucky: We can, theoretically, have multiple orgasms (defined as two or more orgasms separated by a few seconds or minutes with no fading of arousal) or sequential orgasms (defined as a series of climaxes one to ten minutes apart). The reason? Blood flows in and out of a woman's genitals easily, which means that they stay engorged. In contrast, during a man's orgasm, blood flows quickly out of his penis through a network of veins. That's why your guy needs a few minutes (or more) to "recover" after an orgasm before he can get another erection.

While this should *not* become a goal to measure yourself against, 85 percent of the men who answered our survey claim to have witnessed their woman having multiple orgasms. (Of course, 11 percent answered that they weren't sure.) Please note that we did *not* ask them how they knew their lady was having multiple orgasms, nor did we ask them whether it was a good thing or not.

Remember, sex should be pleasure-oriented, not goal-oriented. However, if you'd like to test out your ability to have multiple Os, feel free to experiment by continuing to

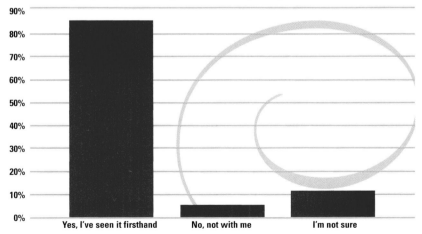

Have any of your partners experienced multiple orgasms?

Have you ever experienced a multiple orgasm yourself?

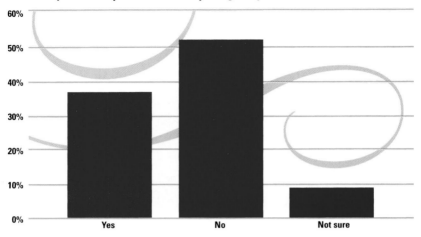

	Yes	No	Not sure

stimulate yourself after your first orgasm. You may need to move to the area surrounding your clitoris, as your love bud itself may be too sensitive for continued direct stimulation. You may still feel overstimulated, but that feeling may transform itself into another round of exquisite pleasure. During partner sex, you can also try varying the type of stimulation you're receiving. For example, change from missionary position to woman on top, or have your man switch from being inside you to massaging your clitoris.

Can men have multiple orgasms? According to our survey, many claim they have, although the majority—53 percent—haven't reached these heights.

Full disclosure time: Our survey didn't ask *how* they achieved multiple orgasms. We suspect that many of our respondents defined "multiple orgasms" as the ability to have another erection as soon as possible after ejaculation and to have another climax. In fact, male multiple orgasm is usually described as the ability to have multiple orgasms

—without ejaculating or losing an erection—until a final orgasm.

Our guess is that they may have experienced an extended or more intense climax rather than a true multiple orgasm. Either way, it's a worthy event. Want to try it? One way is to bring him close to the point of no return— through oral sex, manual stimulation, or controlling your thrusts during vaginal intercourse—and then stop what you're doing for at least ten seconds. Then start up again. But don't stop more than three or four times, or he may not be able to come at all.

Sexual Buffness

Speaking of orgasms (real, unfaked ones), here's a way to have better ones: Do your Kegel exercises. As many men are already aware, a Kegel is what happens when you squeeze your pubococcygeus (PC) muscle, which runs from your pubic bone to your tailbone, surrounding your genitals. (It's the muscle you use to stop the flow of pee.) You can find it by slipping a finger into your vagina and clenching. To strengthen the muscle, simply squeeze and hold for a few seconds, then repeat. That's a Kegel!

Named after the gynecologist who developed them, Kegel exercises have a plethora of sexual benefits. They increase blood flow to the area, thus enhancing lovemaking, whether you're alone or with a partner. In fact, 67 percent of the men who responded to our survey feel that Kegels make sex better. (Sadly, nearly a third—29 percent— don't know what a Kegel is, but that doesn't mean you shouldn't do them.)

A well-toned PC muscle can also increase clitoral sensa-

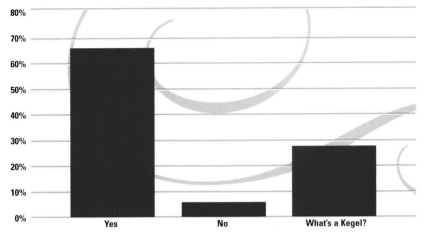

Kegel exercises—do they enhance sex?

tions and vaginal lubrication, produce more intense and stronger orgasms, and help you regain pelvic floor muscle tone after childbirth. Kegels may even help you achieve multiple orgasms. Your man can do Kegels, too; if he does, he may enjoy easier, harder erections and more control over his penis.

Turn-Offs 101

We've talked a lot about what turns men on. When it comes to the act of sex itself, what turns them off? For the guys who responded to our survey, the answer is clear: It's an unenthusiastic partner.

Lack of Interest

If you want to turn your man *off*, here's what you do: Act bored. Lie there passively. Have sex grudgingly. Because there's nothing that will dampen his ardor more than lack of interest. "Obligatory, nonparticipatory sex is the worst and not worth having," says William, 39, a business development manager. Adds T.J., a 42-year-old musician, "Disinterest or 'permission' on her part is a huge turn-off. I only want it if she wants it. Sure, I wish she wanted it every night, but I'm realistic."

So if you're enjoying yourself, let him know. Otherwise, he might interpret your quietness as disinterest. "My biggest turn-offs are a two-way tie between silence (because I get turned on when I can hear her pleasure) and just lying there!" says Patrick, a 40-year-old writer.

Note: Guys want to feel an emotional connection just as much as you do. "My biggest sexual turn-off is when a woman is going through the motions without emotional involvement," says Boris, a 43-year-old creative director. "Or when there's a lack of impulsive interest and desire." Marcus, a 47-year-old manager, comments, "If I feel used, like she's not being interested in me, just my body for sex, that's a big turn-off."

A "get-it-over-with" attitude also cools a man's jets. "I don't like rushing through it," says Bob, a 28-year-old engineer. "I like to just try different things and take some time to discover new things to try and ways to have fun."

Other men cited "women who have hang-ups or guilt issues about sex;" "women who are nonparticipatory or inert;" "a girl who lies like a log with no personality;" "passionless sex;" "when my partner isn't into it;" and "total self-absorption, ignoring me" as major turn-offs.

Lack of Hygiene

The second most common turn-off mentioned by the men in our survey was bad personal hygiene. Guys mentioned body hair, body odor, bad breath, lack of sanitation, and other cleanliness issues (generally centering on excretory functions). So while you don't want to douse yourself in perfume, you might want to avoid garlic and make sure you've showered well before that big date. We won't get more detailed than that.

Distractions

Another turn-off mentioned by several guys is any distraction that takes either of you mentally away from what you're doing. "During sex, nothing should interrupt (excepting emergencies, of course)," says Mike, a 23-year-old restaurant worker and student. "Ignore the phone, forget your self-consciousness and prudery, don't look at the clock." Thirty-one-year-old Clay, an animal control officer, cites "the fact that she could be thinking of anything else but being in the moment" is enough to dampen his ardor.

Other distractions (to him) might even include the environment you create for romance. "If we're that far into it, there aren't many turn-offs," says Simon, 36, a programmer. "The surroundings do matter, though. I can overheat in the blankets that she thinks are just cozy."

Another major distraction? "Work stress," says Alex, a 32-year-old manager. So when your clothes come off, leave the office behind—unless you're getting busy on your desk.

What Comes Out of Her Mouth

Although the majority of men in our survey want you to express your pleasure, they prefer it if you keep your comments (and noises) constructive. "I get turned off by an obsession with simultaneous orgasm, particularly if it's verbalized (i.e., 'Let's come together')," says Robert, a 39-year-old attorney. "It creates too much pressure." David, a 43-year-old systems administrator, cites women who "offer criticism instead of helpful instruction," while George, a 50-year-old attorney, has a problem with "too much talking and demanding."

And while many men like X-rated comments, others, like Ned, a 48-year-old retired attorney, and Scott, a 29-year-old student, find "forced dirty talk" to be a turn-off.

Miscellaneous Turn-Offs

While most of the turn-offs reported by the men in our survey fell into the categories we've just discussed, those weren't the only responses. In fact, the things that turn guys off run the gamut of annoyances, including:

HE SAYS/SHE SAYS

Nima says: For those of you with kids, I empathize, now that we have one of our own. While we love our children, they can be a terrible distraction at best, and a total killer of our sex lives at worst. There's no easy solution, but we suggest making time for sex. I know it sounds prescribed, but making 1:1 time for each other (consider date nights) can actually be wonderfully relaxing and enjoyable—not to mention something you both look forward to!

Cynthia responds: One friend of mine suggested hiring a babysitter or relative to take the kids out (maybe for an overnight sleepover at Grandma's) while you stay home (in bed). Sounds like a good idea to me!

■ ■ ■ ■ ■

Discomforts (of Any Sort)

* "Being in an uncomfortable/awkward position."
  —Dan, 38, real estate agent

* "Fear of getting involved in some kind of trouble afterwards." —Luke, 32, student

HE SAYS

"Let's come together" sounds like one of those ridiculous statements like "learn to control your autonomous nervous system." Get real and just enjoy having your orgasms. Don't pressure yourselves to climax simultaneously.

■ ■ ■ ■ ■

Low Self-Esteem

* "Lack of self-confidence."
  —Tom, 31, attorney

* "Lack of presence." —George, 48, marketing consultant

* "A woman who is not sensual enough, not comfortable with herself."
  —Ted, 44, logistics manager

Lack of Creativity

* "Lack of imagination (even though that sounds corny)."
  —Oliver, 42, educator

* "Having to do it in the bedroom all the time."
  —Ben, 40, architect

Bad Timing

* "If I orgasm before she does." —Kelly, 27, graduate student

And of Course ...

* "Other people nearby." —Pete, 42, sales

* "A bad personality outside the bedroom." —Dave, 41, executive

* "Her going straight to the bathroom afterwards." —Rick, 27, student

Just Do It

Then there are the guys who will persevere in the face of any obstacle. "Nothing has turned me off yet," reports Brian, a 37-year-old entrepreneur. Walt, a 27-year-old marketing manager, asks, "What's my biggest turn-off? I can't think of one."

And for some men, like Dave, a 40-year-old analyst, "not having enough sex" is their biggest turn-off. "Always do it!" he says.

Which brings us back to the key point we've gathered from our survey respondents. When it comes to the act of sexual intercourse, your biggest asset isn't a hot body, the fanciest position, or the coyest lines. It's your genuine enthusiasm for making love with your partner!

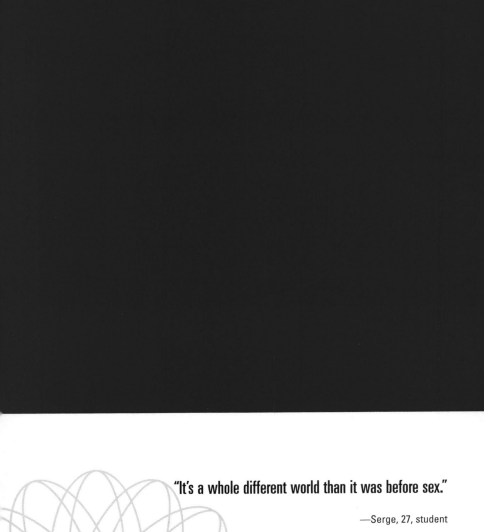

"It's a whole different world than it was before sex."

—Serge, 27, student

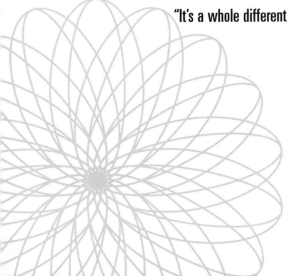

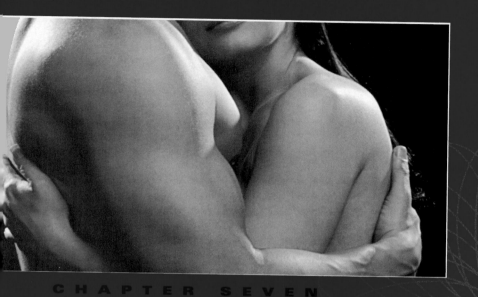

After the Deed

We talked about what happens before and during sex. But what happens after you've knocked boots? Our survey revealed some surprising secrets about postcoital canoodling, as men explained what they wish women knew about cuddling, morning-after turn-ons and turn-offs, why they fall asleep after sex, and what makes them want to run for the door.

The Postcoital Period: What Men Wish Women Knew

If a man had to pick the *one* thing he wished his partner knew about his after-sex state of mind, what would it be? First of all, if he's lying there with half-closed eyes and a smile on his face, for God's sake, *let him be.* Here's why:

 TIP #1: **He's in a state of bliss**

The most frequent word men used to describe their after-sex state of mind was "bliss." As in "I just want to pass out in my state of bliss" (Steve, a 27-year-old student) or "I'm blissed out and usually a little groggy afterwards" (Patrick, a 40-year-old writer). This is good, ladies.

In fact, if it seems that he couldn't string a sentence together to save his life, take it as a compliment. "Usually I don't have full control of my mind after sex," says Jordan, a 45-year-old marketing professional. "I have no politically correct state of mind after sex," says Ted, 27, a production assistant. "I'm worthless." Ned, a 48-year-old retired attorney, puts it more bluntly: "My state of what?"

Don't ruin his blissful state by running out of the room. "Let it linger," says William, a 39-year-old business development manager. "Don't get up immediately and go pee. I like to bathe in the sensuality, smells, and desire of what has just happened." Some men describe the postcoital period in almost religious terms: "It's sacred," says George, 48, a marketing consultant.

And as Serge, a 27-year-old student says, "It's a whole different world than it was before sex."

TIP #2: He's really, really relaxed

HE SAYS

Postcoital bliss leaves us drained—physically, emotionally, and sexually. That after-sex nap is the second-best thing to sex itself.

■ ■ ■ ■ ■

Don't be offended if it seems like your guy is about to fall asleep—or even if he actually does (more on that topic later). The second most common word guys used to describe their state after sex was "relaxed."

"Relaxation and drowsiness do not reflect badly on you," says 42-year-old T.J., a musician. "Quite the opposite. The bigger the orgasm, the longer the recovery time." For stressed-out men, these postcoital moments are precious. "I am *finally* relaxed," says Brian, a 37-year-old entrepreneur. Tom, a 31-year-old attorney, says, "I just want to hang out and relax. Maybe take a nap."

The guys in our survey would like it very much if you chilled out with them after you make love. It's not the time to tackle your chore list. "Let's relax now, please?!" begs Ted, a 44-year-old logistics manager. Peter, a 58-year-old nurse, gets straight to the point: "Relax and enjoy fuck land."

TIP #3: He likes to cuddle (really)

Let's get one thing straight: After sex, "guys like to cuddle, too," as Patrick, a 41-year-old marketing professional, says. In fact, when we asked them, "After-sex cuddling: Yes or no?" a whopping 56 percent of guys answered with a resounding "Absolutely!" Says Dave, a 41-year-old executive, "Nobody really wants to leave if it was really good." Only 5 percent said they wanted to be left alone.

After-sex cuddling: yes or no?

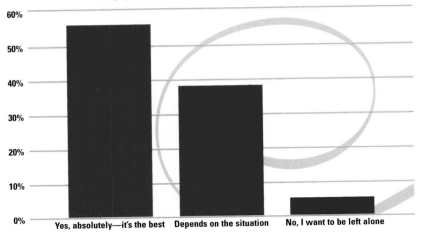

Yes, absolutely—it's the best	Depends on the situation	No, I want to be left alone

For another 39 percent, it all depends on the situation. Some guys are just too wiped out after sex. "We want to relax and cuddle too, but we are very lightheaded and tired (so it's not a bad sign if we feel sleepy)," advises Chris, a 34-year-old software engineer. Others acknowledge the fun of quickies. "It doesn't always have to be the 'spooning/cuddling' thing," says 42-year-old Oliver, an educator. "Sometimes, it's okay to have a 'wham-bam, thank you ma'am' attitude."

If you're lucky enough to find a guy who loves to linger after sex, don't just lie there. "I may not be done and may want to have 'post' play," says 29-year-old Brian, a filmmaker. This could include the "silence, snuggles, smooching" enjoyed by Clay, a 31-year-old animal control officer, or other skin games. "Stroke my chest *reallllly* softly," says Claude, a 34-year-old musician. "It gives me a 'skin-gasm' that induces almost as many groans and shudders as a genital one."

TIP #4: Save the big relationship talk for another time

Yes, you just got physically intimate with your man. That may not, unfortunately, mean that he wants to get *emotionally* intimate. Several guys in our survey echoed the words of

HE SAYS

Shhhhhh, don't talk. It's library time. Please don't act on the urge to say something just to fill in the silence. Snuggle into us and bask in the afterglow that is the bliss of being naked together in bed. We're trying to enjoy our come-drunk stupor.

■ ■ ■ ■ ■

Scott, a 29-year-old student: "It's not the time to have a talk about the relationship." Andy, a 45-year-old electrician, was more direct: "Please don't talk, please don't talk, please!"

That does *not* mean, however, that he's not *feeling* intimate. Chances are he enjoys being with you. He just doesn't want to dissect it verbally. "It's not a very talkative time—and not because I'm not feeling very close to you," says Simon, a 36-year-old programmer. "Just lie with me and look out the window at the moon, you know?" Forty-seven-year-old Marcus, a general manager, agrees: "Men just want to cuddle or sleep after sex—not talk."

Of course, feel free to convey your pleasure at what just happened. "It's important to communicate having enjoyed the experience," advises Randy, a 45-year-old teacher.

TIP #5: He might need a moment before he gets back in the saddle

Let your man catch his breath after you've done the deed. In fact, you might want to keep your hands to yourself for a bit. "After an orgasm, the penis is very sensitive and probably best off left alone," says Mike, a 23-year-old restaurant worker and student. "If you're going for more orgasms, the man will be ready after

HE SAYS

The male penis wasn't designed correctly. The blood we need has to come from somewhere (often the brain), and after we orgasm, it flows back upstairs. By the time it's back, we realize there's a beautiful naked woman next to us, and back it flows to the penis. This whole thing takes a little time, so relax and just enjoy the ride.

■ ■ ■ ■ ■

a short interval. Otherwise, it can kind of hurt."

So give your guy some time. "It takes a while for me to recharge," says Sam, a 52-year-old musician. Mentally, he might be anxious to go another round. His body, however, might not be ready to cooperate, and it could be a while before it is. "I *want* to go again," says Xavier, a 40-year-old engineer.

"Unfortunately, it isn't happening for another hour." Some guys will be raring to go much sooner. "I just need another ten minutes," says 28-year-old Bob, an engineer.

Again, this doesn't mean that all activity has to cease. "First of all, my orgasm doesn't have to be the end," comments Nigel, a 31-year-old scientist. "There are other things we can do to please her until I get hard again. And even if I fall asleep, I like being with her."

But not all guys will fall asleep after sex. "Take some time off and then go back at it," advises Ralph, a 34-year-old graduate student. Or take the advice of J.B., a 50-year-old software engineer: "Once is never enough, but in the interim, hhmmm, yummm, put your head on my shoulder and let's purr and see what comes up."

TIP #6: **He might want to be left alone (but don't take it personally)**

As we mentioned earlier, about 5 percent of our respondents confessed to wanting to be alone after sex. "Leave me alone and let's go to bed," says Bruce, a 31-year-old financial planner. "Let me rest," begs Pete, a

42-year-old salesman. John, a 24-year-old contractor, is blunter about it: "Either leave me alone or give me a blow job so we can do it again."

Don't get upset if your guy wants to retreat alone into his post-sex cave. "Sometimes I just want to get away," explains Matt, a 46-year-old political activist. "It's not a rejection of you."

TIP #7: **It's okay to hang out in bed after sex**

Several guys in our survey professed to being annoyed when a woman leaps out of bed after sex. "Don't go straight to the bathroom," requests Rick, a 27-year-old student.

But other guys showed a little more fastidiousness. "We like to clean up before nodding off or moving on," says 32-year-old Alex, a manager. And that might mean you, too. "Go wipe up!" says Greg, 35, an engineer.

TIP #8: **There's no telling how he'll feel**

And then, there are the guys whose postcoital state of mind didn't fit into any neat category:

* "Remember, when we're done, we're generally done and ready to move on to something else."
  —Joe, 59, consultant

* "My after-sex state depends upon the woman. Some are very needy; others don't relax long enough afterwards and hurry into whatever's next." —Boris, 43, creative director

* "It's *really* different for men, and we can't control that, at least the physical part." —Jack, 52, graphic designer

* "I want Chinese food!!!!" —Ben, 40, architect

The Sleep Question

Women often complain that men fall asleep immediately after sex. (Although, be honest, ladies: We do too sometimes.) There's really no need to be annoyed. Your man is in a very happy place, and every molecule in his body is telling him to nod off. "Biochemically, our body just gave us a powerful sleeping pill, and we're usually fatigued as well, so rest is what feels best," says Richard, a 35-year-old teacher. "After I come, especially if it's multiple times, I'm sleeping," states Allen, a 35-year-old film producer.

Many guys sense that dropping off might not be the most polite thing to do, but they just can't help themselves. As Patrick, the writer, puts it: "I try not to just roll over and sleep, but we do get very grogged out."

Here are some of the reasons your man might start sawing logs after making love:

Sex Is Strenuous (Plus, It's Late)

Intercourse takes a lot out of a man, in more ways than one. Your guy might fall asleep afterwards out of sheer exhaustion:

* "I've just rolled around in bed for forty-five minutes, doing lots of activities, and I've 'deep cycled the battery.'"

    —Malcolm, 34, manager

HE SAYS

I admit, the best sleep is the first thirty minutes you get right after sex. Don't hold it against us.

■ ■ ■ ■ ■

* "I'm damn tired and have been working hard. Sex isn't a passive act for me. I like to make it gymnastic, playful, and active."

    —Bob, 28, engineer

* "We may genuinely be tired, not just faking." —Sam, 46, business consultant

* "Sex can tap all of the energy out of a man." —Sam, 52, musician

* "It takes a lot out of me, and I'm tired (and I've usually just worked a full day)." —Kelly, 27, graduate student

* "1.) We're in bed. 2.) After the sprint to the finish that often occurs in sex, we can be quite tired. 3.) The sheer pleasure afterwards gives me a kind of dreamy euphoria." — Mike, 23, restaurant worker/student

* "Two theories: 1.) I'm tired! 2.) Some single men get in the habit of masturbating right before going to bed, ergo it's conditioning." —Nigel, 31, scientist

More than one guy referred to sex as "hard work" (which makes one wonder how they'd deal with labor and childbirth). "We're the ones who have been doing all the work, typically," says Paul, a 29-year-old graduate student. "If it's been a long session, it's exhausting."

And then, of course, there's the simple fact that men fall asleep after sex "because it's late," as John, the 24-year-old contractor, points out. P.B., a 51-year-old corporate headhunter, elaborates: "It's often late at night, and we're tired. We could have gone to sleep earlier, but we waited to have sex." When you combine the late hour, lots of strenuous activity, and a comfy bed, it's no wonder men doze off. "I always do," admits Brian, the 29-year-old filmmaker. "I'm usually tired by nighttime. After I exert that much energy, I'm usually ready to pass out."

Sex Is Draining

A corollary to the "I fall asleep because sex is strenuous" excuse is the related explanation that sex is just plain "draining," as more than one man termed it. "It takes everything out of us," says Jordan, 45. "It's a very draining experience, literally and figuratively." And some guys do see it in very literal terms: "We lost a bunch of blood to the head and there was exercise involved," says Chris, 34.

Sex Is Relaxing

But no matter what time of day you make love or how much energy you exert, most men admit that they fall asleep afterwards because sex is just so darn relaxing:

* "You're in a wonderful state of relaxation and you just pass out." —William, 39, business development

* "Sometimes you just feel extremely relaxed after a good session with the right woman." —George, 50, attorney

* "Being excited overrides and masks the need for sleep. When that's gone, the sleep urge may take over. Also, it's deeply relaxing and sleep-inducing; we're just wired that way."
  —Sam, 46, business consultant

* "I'm fully satiated and relaxed, and I easily drift into sleep." —Joe, 59, consultant

* "It's natural and we're very relaxed. It's perfect." —Marcus, 47, general manager

* "During orgasm I let everything go, releasing pent-up pressure and causing me to relax. This peaceful relaxation seems to flow into sleep." —J.B., 50, software engineer

* "I feel so relaxed after an orgasm that I can't help but fall asleep." —Walt, 27, marketing manager

* "It's such a high and burst of energy that a lull frequently follows. It's also a relaxing way to fall asleep." —Boris, 43, creative director

Sex Is Satisfying

Another reason is the simple "sense of accomplishment," as Luke, a 32-year-old student, describes it. "If you've had good sex, sometimes you both are so satisfied you fall asleep in fuck land," says 58-year-old Peter, the nurse. "It seems to be a problem if one partner is not quite satisfied."

And Then There's Science ...

For some men, post-sex sleepiness boils down to "nature," according to men like Xavier. Richard, the 35-year-old teacher, gives a more detailed explanation: "Apart from our simply being exhausted from vigorous activity, upon orgasm the gonads release a signal to the brain to bathe in sleep-inducing chemicals, which produce euphoria and hence encourage a sense of attachment."

Or as Ned, 48, puts it so succinctly, "Release, exhaustion, biochemistry."

Pour Me Another Round

If you throw a couple of cocktails into the mix, you increase the chances that your man will nod off after you've done the deed. "Heck, I've fallen asleep *during* sex," says Rob, a 36-year-old sales-

HE SAYS

Ever fall asleep during a massage? Yeah, after-sex sleep can feel like that sometimes. You may not want to, and think it's a bit rude, but oh does it feel good!

■ ■ ■ ■ ■

man. "Generally it's because I'm either drunk or hung over."

Then Again, Sleep Rocks

Of course, as those of us who have children will tell you, don't knock sleep. "It's the next best thing to having sex again," says Bruce, the 31-year-old financial planner.

Want Him to Run for the Door Afterwards? Here's What You Do.

It *is* possible to ruin the afterglow for your guy. Here's how.

Talk Too Much

After a delicious round of lovemaking, resist the urge to fill the silence. One of the most common post-sex turn-offs mentioned by our survey respondents was "talking too much." Some of the subjects men find verboten include discussing work, talking about your ex-lovers, or talking about *his* ex-lovers. "Don't ask me how many people I've slept with," pleads Brian, the filmmaker. "I hate it when someone says, 'That was great, you must have a lot of practice.'"

HE SAYS

My all-time favorite after-sex blow-off comment (from either party) still remains: "It's not you, it's me." Second-place runner-up: "I'd like to date you, but I have to work on myself as a project." What are you, a piece of pottery?

■ ■ ■ ■ ■

As we've noted, it's also not the time to dissect the relationship. Timing is everything. "My after-sex turn-off is talking about what needs improvement (outside of sex) in the relationship," says Sam, the 52-year-old musician, "or bringing up something that should be talked about at a different time." Adds Matt, "It's not the time to say things like, 'Let's talk about us' or 'Where are we heading in this relationship?'"

Most important, getting too talkative takes you out of the moment. "Don't get too chatty," says William. "Let's savor and soak in the sensuality of what we just did."

After sex, it seems, silence truly is golden.

Criticize Him

Remember the old adage, "If you can't say anything nice, don't say anything at all"? Nowhere is this truer than right after sex. Another way to kill the postcoital mood is to criticize his looks, technique, personality, or anything else. "In a committed relationship, my biggest post-sex turn-off is her pointing out flaws in my body or saying hurtful things," says Jordan. "It's a very sensitive time." Randy, the teacher, agrees, saying that it's "communicating that I'm not attractive or sexy." (Do women *really* do this? Yikes!)

Some guys don't want to hear evaluations of any sort. "I hate Monday-morning quarterbacking," says Robert, a 39-year-old attorney. "I don't want to hear effusive compliments. I don't want to be critiqued, either."

Get Clingy

We're sorry to have to tell you this, but getting sweaty and "nekkid" with a guy doesn't automatically make you partners for life. (Don't shoot us: We're only the messengers.) According to the guys who answered our survey, one of their biggest post-sex turn-offs is when you "presume that having sex means more than it actually does," as Paul tells us. "The thing that could get me running for the door is her thinking that sex = marriage = kids," says Mike, the restaurant worker and student. "Of course, I would have tried to find that out beforehand and not had sex with her

HE SAYS

My advice: The best time to talk about relationships and get clingy is after you've had sex at least fifty times, but not before.

■ ■ ■ ■ ■

in the first place."

"Immediately making relationship assumptions is scary, especially if it's the first time we've had sex," agrees Allen, the film producer. Jordan says that while his postcoital turn-offs depend on the situation, "in a noncommitted relationship, it's professing her undying love for me."

So while he may like to cuddle, your guy may need some emotional distance after making love, especially if it's early in the game. Guys like 31-year-old Tom, the attorney, cited "not giving me my space" as one of his biggest turn-offs, while David, a 43-year-old systems administrator, mentioned "pushing too much for a relationship too early."

Now remember, folks, context is everything. If you've been together for a while, expressing your love for each other might be the most natural and appropriate thing in the world. And what better time than after you've actually made love?

What these guys are talking about is pushing for a relationship too soon (like after the first time you have sex), before you've really gotten to know each other. Because guess what? You might not think *he's* such hot stuff after several months. If you tend to get emotionally attached after you've slept with someone, then *wait before you jump into the sack*. And if you do get swept away by passion, don't assume that it means anything more than that you acted on an attraction. Stay in the moment, and protect your heart.

Get Remorseful

The opposite of getting too attached is beating yourself up—*in his presence*—about the fact that you just had sex. Several guys in our survey listed "remorse" on the woman's part as another turn-off. "Don't start feeling guilty or insecure about what we just did, or become upset about something but do the cold-shoulder routine and refuse to talk about it," says Nigel.

"When I was in college, I remember a woman telling me the next morning that 'last night happened too soon,'" says Patrick, the marketing professional. "That was a turn-off. Nothing like having someone regret that they slept with you."

Other guys cited "acting like it didn't happen" (Marcus, 47, general manager); "when she seems uncomfortable with me" (J.B., 50, software engineer); "ignoring the whole situation" (Rick, 27, student); and "talking about the risks of what just happened" (Dave, 41, executive) as major postcoital bummers.

So take responsibility for your actions, ladies. If you wake up and realize you've made a major mistake—like if you had too much to drink and slept with your neighbor, as one of your authors did—wait until he's left before you tear your hair out. Who knows? You might end up marrying him one day, and you wouldn't want him using every cocktail party "How did you guys meet?" query as an opportunity to recount how you could hardly wait to kick him out the door.

Have a Personality Change

Interestingly enough, several men in our survey seem to have gone to bed with one woman, only to wake up with an entirely different—and quite crazy—one the next morning. More than one guy mentioned a woman doing "anything dramatically different from the way she behaved the night before" (Simon, 36, programmer) as enough to turn them off.

"I shudder to think what could get me running for the door," says Richard. "I've never had such an experience and can't imagine what would make me feel that way—apart from a woman acting very differently than she normally does, to the point of suggesting major insanity."

Other guys cited "irrational crankiness or bitchiness" (George, 50, attorney) or "dancing and throwing stuff around the room" (Greg, 35, engineer). T.J. advises caution when it comes to post-sex hilarity, saying he gets turned off "if she gets really giggly and playful right away. Playful is good during sex but not right afterwards. Giggly is never good during or after. Humor is fine, but not giggly."

HE SAYS

Laughter is the best medicine, unless it's right in the middle of the deed. No matter what you say, we're going to think it's about the inadequate size of our penis, and that will pretty much end anything and everything. If you do laugh, cover it up with a clever lie, perhaps something like "(giggle, giggle) I can't believe it took me this long to finally sleep with you. You're fucking great! And your penis is huge!"

■ ■ ■ ■ ■

Light Up a Cigarette

Got a smoking habit? Here's a good reason to quit—it's a big sexual turn-off, according to several men who answered our survey. Ted, the 44-year-old logistics manager, goes so far as to equate it with the sin of "wanting to know what I'm thinking."

Run Off into the Bathroom

Yes, we've already told you that many of the guys who responded to our survey want you to have good habits when it comes to your personal hygiene. However, don't feel like you have to indulge those habits the moment you finish making love. Men like Peter mentioned "getting up right after and taking a shower" as a huge mood-killer. Sex might be messy, but it isn't dirty, and hopefully, neither is he. "Don't run to the bathroom right away to clean up," says Ben, a 40-year-old architect. "Take it easy, relax, and lay there for a while."

If you must bathe after sex, suggest he join you. You might just get him interested in another round. And when you do head off to clean up, be considerate. Andy, the 45-year-old electrician, recounts the time a woman "took the blankets into the shower with her. She was cold."

Go for the Happy Ending

For a certain group of guys, there's basically nothing you could do to kill their postcoital mood. "It hasn't happened yet," says writer Patrick. Meanwhile, Claude "can't think of anything" that would get him running for the door after sex. But we wouldn't suggest pushing a guy too far. Sure, these guys might not mind if you smoked, criticized them, started talking about wedding reception sites, or ran for the shower right after you've had sex with them. But we wouldn't suggest it—unless you've been together for a while.

What are better options? Snuggle into him, bask in the afterglow, and drift off into a postcoital power nap. There's nothing better, and he'll thank you for it.

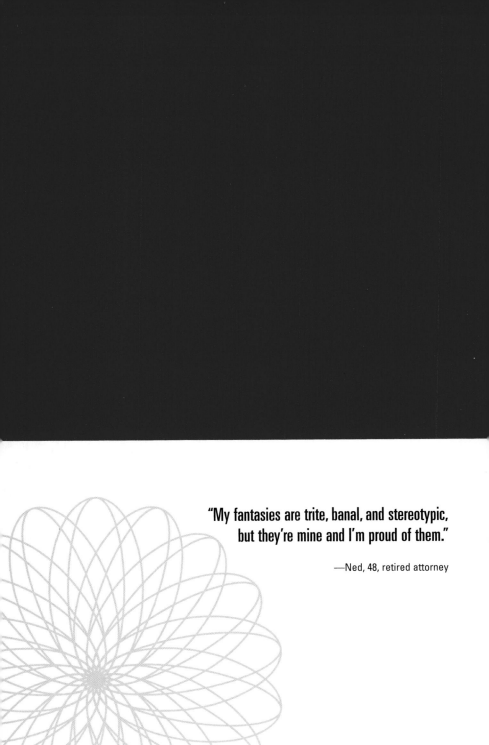

"My fantasies are trite, banal, and stereotypic, but they're mine and I'm proud of them."

—Ned, 48, retired attorney

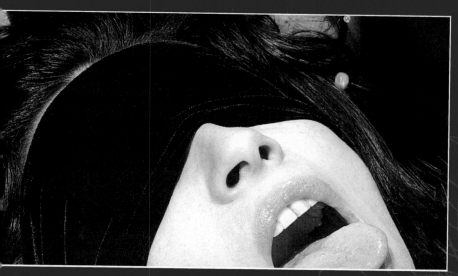

CHAPTER EIGHT

Fantasy Island

You've heard the statistic that men think about sex every few minutes. Assuming that's true, what exactly do they think about? In this chapter, guys give us a glimpse into their secret erotic desires—desires they may not act out, but that turn them on all the same.

His Sexual Fantasies: What Men Wish Women Knew

What does your man wish you understood about his sexual fantasies? Make no mistake, he *does* have them, and that's perfectly healthy. Unfortunately, "most men are taught they're wrong," says 52-year-old Jack, a graphic designer. Sadly, many women are, too. That's a shame, because fantasies can be one of the safest and most enjoyable ways to turn yourself on. Here's what you should know about his:

TIP #1: **He has a lot of them, and that's okay**

First of all, no matter how satisfied your guy is with you, "we do have fantasies," points out Robb, a 59-year-old scientist. In fact, men have "lots of them," according to Gene, a 64-year-old writer.

His fantasies are where he can let his mind run wild. "We fantasize about having sex with all kinds of different women, real and imaginary, because it's safe and fun and not anything we can biologically prevent doing," says Richard, a 35-year-old teacher. "My fantasies are trite, banal, and stereotypic, but they're mine and I'm proud of them," chuckles Ned, a 48-year-old retired attorney.

Keep in mind that while fantasies are a great way for him to channel his sexual energy, they're not a replacement for the real thing. "Fantasizing is just something to occupy my mind while masturbating," notes J.B., a 50-year-old software engineer. "I'd rather be with you." In fact, you may even be the subject of his fantasies. "I've probably already fantasized about doing everything under the sun with her before we actually do it for the first time," says 40-year-old Ben, an architect.

Sexual daydreams can also "help enhance sex and should not be thought of badly," says Chris, 34, a software engineer. Adds Peter, a 58-year-old nurse, "It's just an added dimension to sex."

TIP #2: **Don't be threatened— they're called fantasies for a reason**

HE SAYS

Fantasies are practice for the real deal. They're also sometimes a safe alternative when you're not particularly in the mood or we're not that capable.

■ ■ ■ ■ ■

For most men, fantasies are only that. "Just because you think about them doesn't mean you will go out and do them," says David, a 43-year-old systems administrator. "They're all essentially safe," adds George, 48, a marketing consultant. And no matter how elaborate his fantasies are, "they don't mean I should be in jail," says 35-year-old Greg, an engineer.

Most important, his fantasies don't threaten you. "They're just things that sound good in an ideal world, but we know would be disastrous in the real world," admits Jordan, a 45-year-old marketing professional. "My fantasizing doesn't mean she doesn't already turn me on," says T.J., a 42-year-old musician.

And he might be perfectly content to leave his fantasies in the realm of his imagination. "Acting them out would be fun but not necessary," says T.J. In fact, he may have no wish to see them become real. "They're fantasies ... not necessarily desires," comments Allen, a 35-year-old film producer. Adds Matt, a 46-year-old political activist, "I'm not being disloyal to you when I have these fantasies. I don't necessarily want to act them out with you or anyone else, for that matter."

That's why he may not share them with you. "Women don't need to know what my fantasies are," says Brian, a 29-year-old filmmaker. "That's why they're fantasies. If they

A friend of mine called fantasies "erotic safe havens," partly because he felt free to let his imagination run wild when he had them, and partly because he felt his girlfriend just wouldn't understand if he shared them with her. That's unfortunate, because most fantasies are healthy and probably indicative of a wonderfully imaginative lover.

■ ■ ■ ■ ■

 TIP #3: He'd like to talk about them with you

come true, it's great; if not, they can stay fantasies."

To men, fantasies are healthy fun, whether they're enacted or not. "Just because I have a certain fantasy doesn't mean I want to live it out with her," says 41-year-old Patrick, a marketing professional. "And likewise. It's okay for her to have wild sexual fantasies. I'm not going to be offended if they don't involve me. That's why they're called fantasies."

According to the guys who responded to our survey, men would love to share their fantasies with you—if they could be sure that your reaction would be positive. "I wish they could just enjoy them and play along," says Sam, a 52-year-old musician. "I like to talk about them, and their interest should be supportive," says 34-year-old Claude, another musician. "There should be no threatened feelings on either side."

Most of all, they'd like you to cut them some slack. "It would be okay to simply indulge me," says Rob, a 36-year-old salesman. And with some guys, you won't have to play any guessing games: "The women I've been with *know* all my fantasies," points out Paul, a 29-year-old graduate student.

Remember, in his mind, talking about a fantasy doesn't mean he expects it to happen. Sometimes, just discussing a sexual daydream is erotic enough. "Not every sexual fantasy has to be achieved," says Dave, a 41-year-old executive. "It's okay to fantasize together for a thrill."

On the other hand, he wouldn't mind if you literally made his dreams come true, either. Which brings us to our next tip:

TIP #4: **He might want to try some of his fantasies**

Many of the guys in our survey said that they'd like it—very much—if you tried out some erotic daydreams with them. "I wish women knew how to make my fantasies come true," says 27-year-old Steve, a student. "Take the initiative, or be excited about engaging in some harmless fantasies," suggests Clay, a 31-year-old animal control officer. P.B., a 51-year-old corporate headhunter, urges you to "explore—try new things, wear something different."

Not every guy wants to try everything he daydreams about: "Some are just fantasies, and some would be fun to turn into realities," points out Brian, a 37-year-old entrepreneur. On the other hand, some do. "I will eventually want to try all of them," says 46-year-old Sam, a business consultant.

But make no mistake, ladies: Your guy wants to explore his fantasies with *you*. "You really want to try your fantasies, and it would be better if it's not with a random girl," explains Serge, a 27-year-old student. "I want to live them out with her," adds Rob, a 45-year-old self-employed consultant. Guys know that sometimes, bringing a fantasy to life can truly enhance lovemaking: "When you come together to make do-able fantasies a reality, you can have a good time indeed," comments 41-year-old Patrick, a marketing professional.

Remember, too, that while some guys will be glad to share their fantasies with you, others want to take a more subtle approach and hope you follow their cues. "While common, talking about the fantasy sometimes destroys it," Robert, a 39-year-old attorney, comments. "Some people are shy about articulating their fantasies, so they give hints. And if they do, it can come across as judgmental to verbalize about it ('So you want me to watch you jacking off on me while I'm wearing garters?'). Instead, just do it— put on the garters and tell me to jack off on you; make my fantasy your fantasy; I'll let you know if it's not right. You need to be subtle, creative, and speculative."

 TIP #5: He might be thinking of other people (but that's okay)

This may or may not come as a shock to you, but *very* occasionally, your man might daydream about the latest *Sports Illustrated* swimsuit issue cover model when he's with you. Actually, he may have these daydreams more than occasionally. "I frequently think of other partners," says Joe, a 59-year-old consultant. According to our survey responses, fantasizing about other partners is a common and totally harmless pastime. And let's be honest: You've never thought about someone else when you're in the throes of passion?

And yes, your man may fantasize about other women, but it doesn't mean he's going to cheat on you. Matt sums up the sentiments of most of the guys who answered our survey when he says, "I think you'd think I was

HE SAYS

If we feel comfortable in our relationship, we're more likely to share our fantasies with you. Just don't run away screaming and treat us like lepers if we do.

■ ■ ■ ■ ■

rejecting you if I told you about all the women I think about having sex with every single time I think of them. It's just a thought, almost a reflex, like 'Gee, she has a nice face' only I think, 'I'd like to do her.' I probably really wouldn't, but I like to think about it—kind of like my own free porno movie. I have women friends whom I think about doing all the time, but I won't tell them about it and I won't necessarily tell you."

Your man's fantasies may serve an important purpose when you're not around. "We use them to take care of ourselves when you're not available, so we *are* thinking about you," says Alex, a 32-year-old manager.

 TIP #6: His fantasies run the gamut You may be wondering, what *do* guys fantasize about? The specific fantasies mentioned in our survey were spread across the board. Some were a little wild, while others merely involve you taking the initiative:

* "It usually involves having sex in places or situations I haven't in the past." —Tom, 31, attorney

* "Lesbians are a huge turn-on. I don't get it either, but they *so* are." —Patrick, 40, writer

* "They involve the woman seducing me." —Randy, 45, teacher

* "The only essential recurring element is that the woman is wildly eager to do whatever I think feels good at any given time. Utterly horny, and I get to be lazy: no communication effort required." —Simon, 36, programmer

* "Anal sex adds another dimension." —John, 24, contractor

HE SAYS

Incredibly, not all male fantasies involve a beer in one hand, the remote control in the other, and the woman performing oral sex on him during a football game.

* "I would love to try swinging. I feel secure in my relationship, and I would love to watch my woman with another man or woman." — Walt, 27, marketing manager

* "I don't have that many sexual fantasies." —Kelly, 27, graduate student

* "There is almost nothing I wouldn't try." —Morgan, 27, financial analyst

And some of the things you might think are common male fantasies really aren't. For example, "not all men are into multiple partners," says Dave, a 40-year-old analyst. Fantasies are as individual as the men who have them.

The Pornography Question

No issue strikes as much insecurity into the hearts of women as the pornography question. Why do men like it? (And not all men do.) Does it mean he doesn't find you attractive? Should you look at it with him, or make him throw it out? Even women who have healthy erotica collections of their own can find themselves taken aback when they find their mate's secret stash of *Perfect 10* magazines. Well, ladies, we want to tell you one thing: Chill out.

He Has to Have It

Like it or not, pornography is a staple of the male sexual psyche. Many of the men who responded to our survey were adamant about their need for it, calling it "a necessity" (Luke, 32, student) and "a fact of life" (Bob, 28, engineer) in which men indulge "whether you're married or single" (Steve, 27, student). "We have to have it," says Pete, a 42-year-old salesman, and the sooner you accept that fact, the better. "There's a place for it in our lives—let it be!" says Paul, a 29-year-old graduate student.

HE SAYS/SHE SAYS

Nima says: If his porn really bothers you, get your own. If that bothers *him*, then you can both talk about it. Otherwise, let it be (as long as it's in a place the kids can't get to).

Cynthia responds: Regarding that last comment, know that little boys will naturally be curious about—and will find— their father's porn stash, so choose your off-hours reading carefully.

■ ■ ■ ■ ■

To some men, porn is such an everyday fact of life that it's no big deal. For guys like P.B., the 51-year-old corporate headhunter, an interest in porn is "pretty meaningless." In fact, "we think it's funny," says Andy, a 45-year-old electrician.

Perhaps a tad defensively, many guys took pains to point out that having an interest in pornography was a "perfectly normal" activity. "We've been doing it since we were wee lads, and it's a safe, private, normal, and familiar release for us and has nothing whatsoever to do with them," says Claude, a 34-year-old musician. Adds Marcus, a 47-year-old general manager, "We like it, and it doesn't make us so perverted that we can't live in society like everyone else. We'll still make good husbands and parents."

Some men even suggested that it would be unusual for a man *not* to like pornography (although as we'll discuss in a bit, there are some perfectly normal guys for whom it holds no appeal). "If I'm not interested in looking at beautiful bodies in print, I'm either dead or I'm probably not going to be interested in you either," says Alex, a 32-year-old manager.

Don't Be Threatened by It

Your man's interest in porn doesn't change his feelings for you one bit—at least, that's the assurance we got from our survey respondents. Pornography is "a turn-on but not a replacement," say guys like 34-year-old Chris, a software engineer. "It doesn't take away from how I feel about them," points out George, a 48-year-old marketing consultant. In fact, it may very well *enhance* his desire for you, as Morgan, a 27-year-old financial analyst, comments. "We aren't using it to replace them, and it actually makes us want them more," he says. "I use it to get sexually stimulated, not to fantasize about the girl on the video."

It also doesn't imply that your sex life is lacking. "Just because we might enjoy it, it doesn't mean we think less of you or that you're not fulfilling us," says Ben, a 40-year-old architect. "Don't take it personally!" Nor does it mean your guy expects you to reenact what he sees on film or in print: "It's fantasy," says Brian, a 37-year-old entrepreneur. "I have no expectations for similar actions from my significant other."

More than one man noted that you should keep in mind the fact that porn appeals to men's visual orientation, nothing more. "We think differently," claims Pete, a 51-year-old artist. "Men are visually stimulated, and women tend to be stimulated on more of a mind level." Peter, a 58-year-old nurse, puts it more bluntly: "Men are fascinated by looking at pussies and the sex act." Again, this has nothing to do with you:

* "We're not judging them against the women featured in pornographic images. It's strictly visceral stimulus."
  —Jacques, 52, graphic designer

* "Just because we get wildly turned on by watching other beautiful women having sex doesn't mean we don't enjoy having sex with our mate, nor does it mean we love them any less." —Richard, 35, teacher

* "It's just a visual stimulus. It doesn't hold the same appeal as a real woman and all the other senses that she appeals to." —Jordan, 45, marketing professional

* "It turns me on to see naked women and sexual situations, but it doesn't belittle my feelings toward you." —William, 39, business development

A few guys suggested that porn, by being a safe conduit for their sexual impulses, is a much better pastime than some other activities they could be pursuing. "Just as sports allow violence to be channeled into a safer venue, so pornography allows the biological male tendency toward promiscuity to have an entirely fictional outlet," says Richard. (We think this is a bit sexist—we're not sure that men are programmed for promiscuity—but, who knows, he may have a point.)

David, a 43-year-old systems administrator, reminds us that an interest in porn does *not* mean he's unfaithful: "Every man has at least a passing curiosity about it. It's not a big deal. It's better to masturbate to some image in a magazine or video than to go out and engage in risky sex with a stranger." (He may have a point, too, but we'll also assure you that most guys won't go out and cheat on you if they can't get their hands on a copy of *Hustler*.)

Bottom line: There are other things to get stressed about. Ned, a 48-year-old retired attorney, may sum it up best when he says, "It's like eating Frosted Flakes. Some men do, some men don't, and some men like it really, really a lot. Whatever. In the end, it doesn't cause any significant harm, so stop worrying about it!"

Caveat: If your guy's interest in porn seems to be crowding out all other activities—you know, like eating or sleeping or having sex with his significant other—or seems to veer toward practices charitably described as illegal, then all bets are off. We could get into a whole discussion here about what's "normal" or not, but our guess is that you know where to draw the line.

He Wants You to Enjoy It with Him

There's only one thing better than being understanding about your man's interest in pornography—and that's enjoying it with him. "We *all* read it, stash it away somewhere, and love it; so if you can embrace that and not make him feel like a perv, your man will love you for it!" says Patrick, a 40-year-old writer. Furthermore, "guys are not going to think less of a woman for liking it," says Walt, a 27-year-old marketing manager. "In fact, it's a huge turn-on when a woman is into porn." For many men, watching pornography together can serve as foreplay:

* "Don't feel like you are in competition with it. In fact, if you're into it, that's a definite plus. Even better if you watch with me." —Mike, 23, restaurant worker/student

* "Porn is a good thing, and women shouldn't be intimidated by it. (By the way, my definition of porn can be anything from soft-style erotic stories to hard-core video.)

Experiencing porn together can make for a fun play night." —Patrick, 41, marketing professional

* "It'd be cool to watch with the right woman." —Ted, 27, production assistant

* "Men like it and really would like their partners to enjoy it with them." —Sam, 52, musician

But some guys may *not* want to watch it with you because they don't want to deal with the possibility that you'll judge them. "I like porn a lot, but I don't necessarily want to watch it with you because I think you'll be turned off by it and think it is degrading to women or just plain stupid and gross," says Matt, a 46-year-old political activist.

Above all, if you're going to have an X-rated video night with your guy, keep your insecurities in check. Advises Robert, a 39-year-old attorney, "If you're going to do it with me, don't ask a bunch of comparative questions like, 'Do you think she's pretty?' 'Do you like big, small, medium, etc.?' 'Is she prettier than I am?' I'm not comparing the women on-screen with you, so it's a huge turn-off when *you* do it."

It's a Chance to Learn Something about Him

Another reason you might want to greet your man's suggestion that you watch porn together with an enthusiastic "I'll pop the popcorn!": It's an almost unrivaled opportunity to get a glimpse into his psyche. "Looking at your man's porn collection can help

HE SAYS

That's why *Playboy* is so great. It's got articles for you, pictures for him!

■ ■ ■ ■ ■

you figure out what his turn-ons are," says Nigel, a 31-year-old scientist. Thirty-six-year-old Simon, a programmer, compares porn to junk food. "Smart people mostly avoid it, but I'd wonder about any man who didn't find it compelling," he says. "It's stupid, but it's designed to press our buttons, and it does. If you want to learn how to press our buttons, you might learn something from it."

That's why you should be careful about passing judgment about what you're seeing. "If you don't like it, let him know, but also realize you are missing something about his sexuality," says 34-year-old Malcolm, a manager. A better approach might be to ask him—at a later time and in a nonjudgmental manner—what appealed to him about that particular video or picture.

In fact, while you don't want to overanalyze his interest in plot lines that center around—oh, say, smearing peanut butter over body parts—subtle, curious questions about what you're seeing might yield interesting answers. For example: "I actually like classic porn with stories and women in clothes and a plot line, not just naked people having sex," says Matt. "I like older women–younger men sex fantasies, but that doesn't mean I want to have sex with my mother. I like it when the women appear to be having a good time in the movies, because I hate the thought of them being coerced into having sex on film. I don't want to watch porn that is violent. I like voyeur stuff, and I like to think the stuff that looks real is really faked because it does creep me out if it is real."

Ask your man what he likes and why (and don't be shocked by whatever he tells you). If he's reticent, tell him what turns *you* on about what you've just seen. Chances are, you'll soon be reenacting a couple of choice scenes.

It Can Be Good for Your Sex Life

Which brings us to our next point: Porn can be good for your lovemaking, according to several guys who answered our survey. By stimulating your imagination, "it can act as a fun stimulator and a source of variety," points out Oliver, a 42-year-old educator. Some men even think it makes them better lovers. "Without it, we wouldn't be able to please them as well, and we would bother them a whole lot more," says John, 24, a contractor.

Some Guys Aren't into It

Yes, they do exist: men who are *not* interested in pornography. "We're not necessarily *all* into the stuff," Ted, a 44-year-old logistics manager, assures us. For some, porn is just too obvious. "Explicit isn't always interesting," says Boris, a 43-year-old creative director. "Subtle is intriguing."

But the most common reason men gave is that quite simply, they prefer reality. "The real thing is always better," says Sam, a 46-year-old business consultant. "Who cares about pictures?" Brian, a 29-year-old filmmaker, asserts. "I'm one of the few guys who does not watch porn, has never looked at porn on the Internet, and does not look at magazines. I don't dislike porn; I just like the real thing better."

As J.B., a 50-year-old software engineer, sums it up: "I'd rather be with you."

Sex, Lies, and Videotape

There's watching someone else have sex on-screen or in a magazine—and then there's starring in your very own hard-core movie. Of the men we surveyed, 33 percent had—with their partner's permission—taken a picture of or videotaped themselves having sex. Some, like Paul, a 29-year-old graduate student, did it "just out of curiosity." Others found it to be a real thrill, during and after the relationship (which could be a good reason for *not* doing it). "It's great, even after the relationship is over," says Malcolm, a 34-year-old manager. Claude, a musician of the same age, feels that although "it's weird to watch years later after you've broken up, it's pretty hot, especially while masturbating."

Several of the guys found the experience to be pretty darn erotic. "In my boss's office after-hours, we did a corny little 'fake' porno where she was being interviewed by me

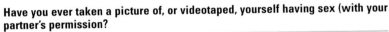

Have you ever taken a picture of, or videotaped, yourself having sex (with your partner's permission?

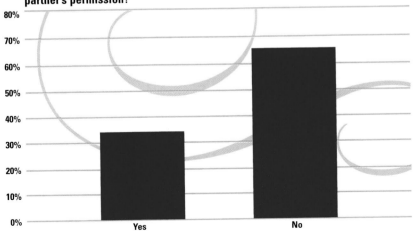

182

for a job," recounts Morgan, a 27-year-old financial analyst. "I was so excited and nervous that I came early." The sense of danger heightens the thrill: "Making a video of yourself is always dangerous to do, but a turn-on both when you do it and when you watch it later," says Marcus, a 47-year-old general manager. In fact, "the act of doing it was better than watching it afterwards," says Jack, a 52-year-old graphic designer.

However, the majority of guys—66 percent—haven't committed their sexual exploits to film. These men fell into two camps. In the first were the men whose interest was tempered by reality. "It could be fun, but it doesn't interest me enough to actually try it," says 46-year-old Sam, a business consultant, "because then you have a stupid-looking tape of yourself being clumsy and overweight." For others, the risk outweighs the potential for titillation: "I've taken naked pictures," says Nigel, a 31-year-old scientist. "But filming sex, no. There's *way* too much risk for all parties. Breakups happen, people run for office, etc." Allen, a 35-year-old film producer who perhaps knows what he's talking about, advises, "This *always* comes back to haunt you."

In the second camp were the guys who would jump at the chance to film themselves in compromising positions. "I would love to try it, but never had a partner who was interested," says J.B., a 50-year-old software engineer. "The idea turns me on," says 40-year-old Patrick, a writer.

I'm Ready for My Close-Up: Sexual Role-Playing

There's a reason that Halloween is such a popular holiday for children *and* adults: It gives us a socially acceptable excuse to play at being someone else. The same holds true

183

in the bedroom. Taking on a temporary role with your lover—sultan/harem girl, stern teacher/eager pupil, goddess/devotee—can add spontaneity and playfulness to your relationship. For many men, role-playing gives them a chance to bring their hottest fantasies to life, which might be why 45 percent of the men in our survey said "Sure, why not?" when we asked them if they had any interest in trying it.

Even men who might not suggest it are open to the idea. "It's not something I'd initiate, but it could certainly spice things up," says Ted, a 27-year-old production assistant. "Variety adds novelty, which makes sex more exciting," says Dan, a 38-year-old real estate agent, "and role-playing lets you express arousing fantasies." Role-playing is also a way to "challenge the safe confines of a predictable sexual relationship," according to Malcolm, a 34-year-old manager.

Role-playing can be a safe way to explore fantasies while giving your erotic imagination free rein. "I think it lets us expand our sexual repertoire in a safe way because you're taking on a role," says Jordan, a 45-year-old marketing professional. "It's not really you, just someone you play. That way I can try being a dom, a sub, a teacher, or a student, without taking that on as part of my persona." Some men saw this aspect less positively. People engage in role-playing because they "are neither satisfied with who they are nor who they are with," claims 45-year-old Randy, a teacher.

But for the men who've tried it, role-playing can open up new sexual vistas. "I've tried some very mild role-playing," says Dan. "We didn't get into full character. It was just comments and attitudes. She was the whore or little girl, me the daddy, or things like that. It was excellent and added to the arousal."

It can also be a lot of fun: "My girlfriend and I once attended one of those dinner games where everyone dresses in costume and solves a mystery," says Patrick, a 40-year-old writer. "I was a roguish Aussie tracker and she was a straitlaced English archeologist. We had such a great time! Now she loves it when I whisper to her in my Australian accent. It almost always leads to sex. It's just a lot of fun and it definitely enhances sex."

Other men have taken role-playing much further. Thirty-four-year-old Malcolm describes experiences that were "planned with costumes, hotel rooms, and different cities. Others have been exploits at work, churches, or parents' houses. In general, the experiences were enjoyable, fun, and satisfying. They enabled different types of interactions, like having sex with clothes partially on or ripped-off, or in positions of submission."

Turn-on or Turn-off?

For one-third of our survey respondents, role-playing holds no interest. These men find reality sexy enough. "I've been encouraged by different partners to play roles or accept their roles," recounts Randy. "I think I was once asked to play doctor and give an examination. It didn't work for me. I like being me and for my partners to be themselves, although I do enjoy their nastier, wilder selves. I like sex to be real, rather than fantasy." David, a 43-year-old systems administrator, says, "I'm not against the idea, but I usually believe in living for the moment and 'loving the one you're with.'" Adds Ted, the 27-year-old production assistant, "I'm not big into role-playing in general outside of the bedroom, so I'd need someone else to really want me to do it."

And some men equate role-playing with the waning of a sexual relationship. "I guess I've just never got to the point of boredom in bed where I ask myself 'What can we do now?' and go down the fantasy/role-play road," says Paul, a 29-year-old graduate student.

For 21 percent of our survey respondents, their interest in role-playing depends on their partner and the situation—namely, how safe they feel in the relationship. "You have to feel safe with that person, both emotionally and physically," Jordan says. "I never felt safe with my last girlfriend, so I never explored anything. It's also why I never slept well when I was with her." Patrick, the writer, agrees. "A lot of guys get self-conscious, so you really have to trust that your partner won't laugh at you or get turned off," he says.

For some men, it relates to how established the relationship is. "I'd only do it to keep things moving—if it's role-playing or nothing," Ted, the 27-year-old production assistant, says. "That would mean it's probably already a longtime relationship, or perhaps a first-time/first-night relationship. I feel like it would be less likely in a young but existing relationship."

Sometimes it simply depends on the two people involved. "Some partners are capable of constructing the illusion and environment for role-playing,"

HE SAYS

Props and role-playing can be healthy ways to act out some of our fantasies with you. But most of the time, we'll only do it if we feel comfortable with you. Handcuffs, for example, are really more about trust between partners than control.

■ ■ ■ ■ ■

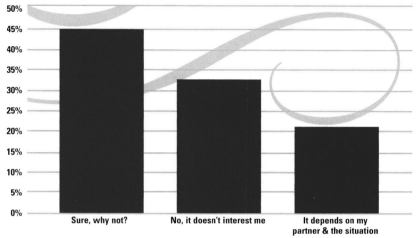

Any interest in sexual role-playing?

| | Sure, why not? | No, it doesn't interest me | It depends on my partner & the situation |

says Malcolm. "Others just can't keep a straight face."

Other men see it as a way to escape reality—but not in a positive way. "Some guys choose to have sex with partners that they're not particularly sexually attracted to," claims Randy. "Role-playing enables them to be whomever they are not and be with someone who's not there."

We tend to see role-playing more benignly. Dressing up as someone else—or simply pretending to be a character—can get you in the mood and, in a safe relationship, let you explore aspects of your sexual personality that you might otherwise repress. It's called role *playing* for a reason.

Beyond Vanilla: BDSM

Kinkiness: It's in the eye (or mind) of the beholder, especially when it comes to practices like bondage and discipline, dominance and submission, and sadomasochism—

known collectively by the acronym BDSM. Contrary to popular belief, you don't have to own leather or like to be whipped to play at BDSM. You just have to be willing to push your boundaries and explore new, possibly unsettling sensations (which is why it works best in a well-established relationship where there's a lot of trust).

Still, the men in our survey were divided about the appeal of BDSM. Twenty-nine percent were willing to try it "as long as no one gets hurt." For these men, BDSM allows them to relinquish (or accept) control, and yes, get closer to their partners.

* "I have a strong domination streak and want to role-play where the woman gives up all control and I own her mind and body." —William, 39, business development

* "There are many, many things I'm willing and eager to try. Mostly, I like a woman who dominates and is rough." —Mike, 23, restaurant worker/student

* "I like to be dominated, which I'm usually pretty open about early on. It keeps two bottoms from getting stuck together." —Nigel, 31, scientist

* "I've tried handcuffs and 'rough' sex. It was awesome, and both of us liked it a lot. Different reasons for her, but for me, it was control and the sharing of intimate fantasies that was so great." —Dan, 38, real estate agent

* "The appeal is the loss of control—having to give up all control to someone else. It's a new side of me. On the flip side, it's about pushing your lover to the edge and pulling her back. For me, it's about seeing how much ecstasy you

can give your lover." —Jordan, 45, marketing professional

* "Tying up your girlfriend is fun—and so is getting tied up by her! It's great having someone completely at your mercy. We bought some fur-lined handcuffs and tied them to the corners of the bed. Now anytime we get into a tickle fight, there's an excellent chance one of us will wind up in the cuffs." —Patrick, 40, writer

* "Never engaged in it myself, other than getting flogged at a street fair.

    I did find the experience oddly exhilarating. Once you've had a severe beating, hassles at work the next day seem like nothing in comparison." —David, 43, systems administrator

Pleasure or Pain?

The men who have engaged in BDSM play often described the experience as "intense." Jordan recalls an experience with light bondage: "It was great foreplay. She had to let go and trust me to take her higher. When the roles were reversed, I had to let go and receive, something I don't often do. It really did make things hotter when we got down to the lovemaking because the foreplay had been so intense." Randy, the teacher, described a girlfriend who enjoyed bondage. "I would tie her to the bed with scarves, and her orgasms were the most intense of her life. There was something about her lack of freedom that enabled her to lose the control that otherwise prevented full-blown orgasms. I tried it but didn't enjoy my lack of freedom— although my orgasms were equally intense."

Some guys have tried almost everything, with varying results: "The basics were covered—sex while being tied up, 'dog walking' with a leash, wrestling, striking, hot wax/ice cubes, smacking, golden showers, etc.," says 34-year-old Malcolm, a manager. "The experiences were much more hit-or-miss from a fulfillment perspective. It was also hard to understand who was getting more out of the engagement—the person in control or the person being subdued."

But BDSM holds no interest for nearly 40 percent of our survey respondents, especially those who equate it with hurting someone. "I'm not a big fan of the violent stuff," says Ted. Malcolm agreed: "Quite honestly, when asked to beat my partner in the face, I lost interest."

Says Randy: "Pleasure is pleasure. Pain is pain. To me, the line is clear. Bondage is still a form of pain (withholding freedom), and I derive no pleasure from either giving or receiving pain. But for some people, pleasure and pain responses are closely related. I personally believe BDSM enthusiasts are missing the point."

A Level of Trust

For 32 percent of the men in our survey, their willingness to experiment with BDSM depends completely on their partner and the situation—specifically, how secure they feel in the relationship. "You have to be comfortable enough to 'go for it,' or you might be more embarrassed than turned on," says Dan. Jordan notes, "Again, it's all about trust and feeling safe."

For some men, it can be appealing one day and not the next: "Occasionally, I'm just not in the mood for rough-housing," says Patrick, the writer. "It's easy to get carried away with the rambunctiousness, so you have to watch it or you can get hurt."

It also depends on the psychological makeup of the two people involved, as Malcolm points out: "Some partners are capable of constructing the illusion required for BDSM. Others just can't take the pain or associate pain and pleasure. I also think that there is a stronger connection to emotional or psychological capacities when engaged in BDSM. There is a much larger variation in people at the psychological level. A lot might come out from previous negative experiences like rape, abuse, and neglect, and these will end any sexual relationship (or explain extreme sexual behavior)."

And on the flip side (and we wouldn't be fair if we didn't present the flip side), men like Randy see BDSM as the sign of a doomed relationship and feel that it epitomizes

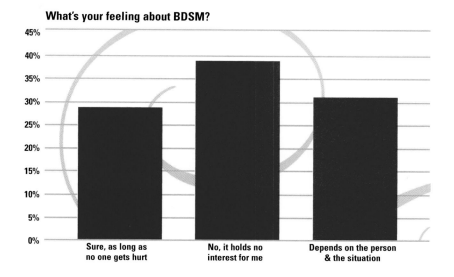

What's your feeling about BDSM?

HE SAYS

For a lot of men, BDSM is a fun way to explore our relationships further and try out a few new things, but it's not really the main course. Once in a while, that kinky spark ignites and we want to be the aggressor, while other times we're perfectly content letting you take control. As with all things, it's important to find out whether these fantasies and role-playing games are a "need to have" or a "nice to have" in your relationship.

■ ■ ■ ■ ■

gender roles. "Once again, many men choose partners who don't sexually arouse them," he says. (They do? That's news to us ... but then, when we think about some of the couples we know, maybe not.) "They search for any role-playing or fantasy situation that might re-spark arousal. In addition, most men are raised with a strong 'man = sadomasochist' background. We are supposed to enjoy a little pain and suffering. That's what being a man is. If we empathize with others and are disturbed by pain and suffering, we're thought of as feminine and weak. Men also confuse dominance with pleasure. Think about the concept of winning."

To some extent, we'd have to disagree. Yes, men in our culture are encouraged toward violence. (Why, we'd like to know, is violence so acceptable on television and in film, but show sex and you're slapped with an NC-17 rating or worse?) But pushing your erotic envelope with BDSM and role-playing is a way to explore your innermost desires and, in the context of an established relationship, stave off predictability (which often *is* the death knell of eroticism). Trying new things together—whether it's a new food or a new sexual game—can take you back to a time when your relationship was new, unknown, and tremendously exciting. Role-playing and BDSM aren't for everyone. But if you're curious and adventurous, go for it—and don't feel guilty!

"Don't be afraid to tell us what really turns you on or what you're into. A lot of us will do anything to please a woman."

—Mike, 23, restaurant worker and student

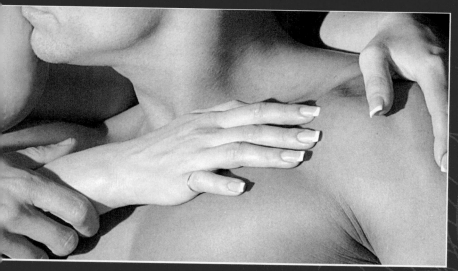

CHAPTER NINE

How to Find Out What <u>Your</u> Man Wants in Bed

In the end, our survey revealed something that we all know, but often forget: While men have some common likes and dislikes, every man has his own specific sexual preferences, quirks, and hot buttons. The only way you're going to find out what your man really wants is to talk to him. He doesn't have ESP, and neither do you. (Oh, you may think you do, but trust us: It's better not to take the chance.)

Kick-Starting the Conversation

Now, when we say you should talk to your man about sex, we don't mean that you should show up on the first date with a list of fifty questions about his sexual preferences. No one likes being grilled (unless it's part of some X-rated detective-suspect role-playing scenario and you're both getting off on it, in which case, you go, girl). We're thinking more of conversations that happen gradually, organically, as you get to know each other and your bodies. Even if it's the first time you're in bed together, you can indicate what you like with words and moans. Here are five tips to get you started:

 TIP #1: **Engage in aural sex** If you're shy about expressing yourself in bed—don't be. Guys love to hear sighs, moans, and cries of ecstasy. (It reassures them that they're doing something right.) Besides, if you hold back on the heavy breathing, you may repress the power of your orgasm. Listening to him will give you a map of what he finds pleasurable, too.

 TIP #2: **Speak up** Just *tell* him you want him to move a little to the left or go faster or slow down or whatever. You don't need to be a drill sergeant. Don't criticize him, either. Gentle coaching works wonders. So next time you're in bed, tell your man at least one thing you'd like him to do. Even if you have been together for ages and aren't particularly shy about sex, it's good practice to ask for something new. We all get into sexual ruts where we assume our partner "just knows" what to do. It never hurts to shake things up.

 TIP #3: **Start foreplay early**   Talk about sex when you're nowhere near a bedroom. Initiate a conversation about sex over a meal or coffee. Be matter-of-fact. Be curious. Use this book as a starting point, if you want. "I read the other day in this great book that 82 percent of men love to watch a woman masturbate. Why do you think that is?" Ask him about his experiences and preferences. You'll not only learn something about him, but, no matter how calm the discussion, you'll get him thinking about what *you'd* look like engaging in whatever practice is under discussion. (Of course, make sure that he's someone with whom you want to engage in that particular practice.) Anticipation can be a huge aphrodisiac, and besides, as we've mentioned, 99 percent of sex happens in the organ between your ears.

It also might be better to talk about sexual problems or issues in a locale other than the bedroom, at a time when you're feeling relaxed. Giving yourselves some distance from "the scene of the crime" may feel safer to both of you.

As the guys in our survey pointed out, the postcoital period is not the time for analyzing his performance or having deep talks about the relationship.

HE SAYS

Taste, touch, smell, sight, and hearing. Our five senses are wonderful avenues to explore during foreplay.

■ ■ ■ ■ ■

HE SAYS

I knew Cynthia would slip this one in. Yes, you can plan not to have sex. However, when you're in bed staring at each other awkwardly because you don't know what to talk about, you can throw this idea out the window and just get it on!

 TIP #4: **Decide not to have sex**

Here's the drill: Each of you gets an entire hour in bed to spend however you choose. The catch: You can't have sex of any type. You can give each other massages or choose to spend the entire hour talking about your day. Although it may seem counterintuitive, deciding consciously *not* to have sex forces you to relate to each other in other ways. You'll feel closer—and that makes for better sex the next time you make love.

 TIP #5: **Share a fantasy**

A survey by the august Kinsey Institute found that 70 percent of men and women have fantasized during sex with a partner. Try sharing one of your fantasies with your mate. (If it's a new relationship, you might want to start with a tamer fantasy.) Gauge his reaction. He'll very likely find the fact that you have such erotic daydreams to be an incredible turn-on.

Then, ask him to share one of his fantasies. You have to promise him, however, that you won't be shocked (or you won't show him that you are).

HE SAYS

Do *not* be shocked if your guy fantasizes during sex. It's totally normal, and many times it's how we control the timing of our own orgasm. *What?!* Yes, we sometimes use fantasies to speed up or slow down the pace of our own coitus so we can last longer or time our own orgasm closer to yours. We fantasize for your pleasure. That's our story, and we're sticking to it.

Don't feel that you're going to have to act out your fantasies unless you want to. Simply describing your sexual thoughts to him can be extremely arousing for both of you. In many ways, revealing what goes on in your head is even more intimate than revealing your body. It can bring you closer and make sex, when you do have it, even better.

Men Give Us Their Parting Shots

We could talk about the topic of sex—and so could the men who responded to our survey—for another 700 pages. Even after answering more than fifty survey questions, some guys had more advice to give. When asked if there was anything else they wanted women to know, they gave us a few choice comments:

Be Enthusiastic

* "I've said this before, but enthusiasm is the most important thing to me. All the other techniques, trappings, and settings, etc. aren't nearly as important as enthusiasm. Besides, when there's enthusiasm, those other things fall into place." —T.J., 42, musician

* "You have got to want it, and show that you want it from me, specifically. Eye contact is vital. I want her to love my come. Inside her or in her mouth. Saying 'mmm' and smiling after swallowing can be hot." —Serge, 27, student

Enjoy Yourself

* "Let go completely. Sex is about just being in that moment, and time and nothing else matters. Don't let anything else

(stress, work, etc.) intrude." —William, 39, business development

* "Life is too short not to enjoy this aspect of our lives."
  —Allen, 35, film producer

Have Confidence in Yourself

* "In general: open, uninhibited, confident equals the best sex." —Nigel, 31, scientist

* "It's okay to be aggressive and make the first move. You can use me as your fuck toy. I don't care."
  —Ben, 40, architect

Connection Is Important

* "For me the key to great sex is a partner who is flexible (both physically and emotionally) and with whom I share a sense of connection." —Sam, 46, business consultant

* "It's not just about sex. It's just that sex makes all the rest much better." —J.B., 50, software engineer

They Don't Always Have to Have Sex

* "Guys don't necessarily have to orgasm to thoroughly enjoy it." —Dan, 38, real estate agent

* "Believe it or not, there really are times when I'm happy to be naked in bed and *not* have sex; well, maybe in a little while ..." —Ted, 44, logistics manager

Watch Your Mental Game

* "Sex is mostly mental. You can put yourself in the mood to have sex just as easy as you put yourself out of the mood." —John, 24, contractor

* "De-emphasize sex as an indicator of love and as validation for your own personal worth." —George, 50, attorney

Looking Does Not Equal Infidelity

* "I can look at other women and still be totally in love with her." —Pete, 51, artist

Fantasizing about Infidelity

* "I wish that having sex with other people while in a committed relationship wasn't so fraught with emotional damage. I'd kind of like the variety, but I know that even if I went off with someone new, after a while I'd still want someone different; I just like novelty and the thrill of the flirting. But being committed is worth more to me than the sexual novelty of a new person. In some ways, I understand when after an affair, the guy says, 'It was just sex! It didn't mean anything!' I know that that isn't acceptable, so I masturbate and fantasize. That's fine with me." Matt, 46, political activist

When it comes to discussing sex, the potential topics are endless.

HE SAYS

Just remember that masturbation is *not* infidelity. We're just practicing our timing and rhythm. Seriously.

■ ■ ■ ■ ■

Closing Words of Wisdom

If there was one thing that came up over and over again in our survey and conversations, it was how much men *want* to talk to their partners about sex. When we told guys we were writing this book, their eyes lit up. They *wanted* to participate in the survey—heck, they wanted all their *friends* to participate in the survey—and they wanted to express themselves. They had tons of opinions and feelings about sex, but no one had ever asked them to share them.

And just as important, they were willing to listen, too. "Women have to be open with men about their sexual desires," says Marcus, a 47-year-old general manager. "There's nothing better than having a meeting of sexual minds!" Adds Mike, a 23-year-old restaurant worker and student, "Don't be afraid to tell us what really turns you on or what you're into. A lot of us will do anything to please a woman."

And be honest. As one man said, "Don't use sex as currency. If you're attracted to someone, show it! We respect your desire more than playing hard to get."

Our culture is sex-obsessed. But while we may leer, we may not appreciate or understand. You can find depictions of every

HE SAYS

Cynthia and I sincerely hope that we've been able to give you a revealing glimpse into the male sexual psyche, and perhaps help you understand us a little better. Ultimately, all men hope that you can look beyond our many faults and sleep with us anyway. If not for love or self-gratification, then at least to ensure the future of the human race. Besides, think how grateful your guy is going to be when you acknowledge his vast porn collection *and* let him keep it!

■ ■ ■ ■ ■

sexual practice under the sun on the Internet, yet many guys remain clueless about how to give their own girl-friend or wife an orgasm. Real discussions about sex remain in short supply. "Our society doesn't make it easy to talk about sex," says 34-year-old Malcolm. "So keep trying!"

Because that's all you can do when it comes to sex: Keep trying. Keep exploring. Keep talking to each other. And most of all, keep on enjoying the sex, and each other!

Acknowledgments

We started this endeavor before the birth of our son and cele-
brated its completion on his six-month birthday. The stress of
work, school, and raising a newborn would have surely over-
whelmed us if it weren't for the love and support of our fami-
lies. We give a heartfelt thanks to Gerry, Michael and Ozi,
Naseem, Rick and Virma, and Jim.

We would also like to thank all the men who responded to
our survey, shared their personal insights and experiences
into the male sexual psyche, answered numerous follow-up
questions, and provided us with the material to write this
book. A special thank you goes to the men and women of the
2006 graduating class of the University of California at
Berkeley's Haas School of Business. And Cynthia would like to
express her gratitude to the women of Word of Mouth Bay
Area for their moral support, and to Leonor, Susan, and Ivana,
for their wonderful, nurturing babysitting services.

Last but certainly not least, we want to thank our agent,
Sheree Bykofsky of Sheree Bykofsky Associates; our publisher,
Holly Schmidt; our editor, Ellen Phillips; and our copy editor,
Amy Kovalski. Their endless patience, unerring guidance, and
thoughtful editing helped bring this book to fruition.

About the Authors

An award-winning fiction writer and screenwriter who self-published her first book of short stories at the age of nine, **Cynthia W. Gentry** is author of *Mind-Blowing Orgasms Every Day: 365 Wild and Wicked Ways to Revitalize Your Sex Life* (Quiver). She is the coauthor, with David Ramsdale, of *Red Hot Tantra: Erotic Secrets of Red Tantra for Intimate Soul-to-Soul Ecstatic, Enlightened Orgasms* (Quiver), for which she wrote the erotica. She also contributed the essay "Following Anaïs" to the anthology *Herstory: What I Learned in My Bathtub...and More: True Stories on Life, Love, and Other Inconveniences* (Adams Media). Gentry has a master's degree in journalism from the University of California at Berkeley, and a bachelor of arts degree in English from Stanford University.

Nima Badiey is a management consultant, avid photographer, and enthusiastic participant in Cynthia's book research. He has masters degrees from the University of California at Berkeley and Stanford University, and a bachelor's degree from University of California, Los Angeles.

Cynthia and Nima live in the San Francisco Bay area with their son.

Index

aggression, 56–57
anal sex, 128
attitude, negative, 54–55, 68–69
aural sex, 88, 116, 132–33, 196

bad breath, 56
bathroom issues, 56
bathroom trips, 164–65
BDSM (bondage, discipline, dominance, submission, sadomasochism), 187–93
bedrooms, 129–30
bikini-line grooming, 61–62, 89
blissful state, 150–51
blow jobs. See oral sex
body contact, 25–27
body parts, sexiest, 29–33
bondage and discipline, 187–93
breasts, 32, 124
butts, 29–32, 121–23

chemistry, 36–37
cigarettes, 164
cleanliness, 55–56, 88–89, 143–44
climax. See orgasms
clinginess, 161–62
clothing, 34–35
communication
    direct, 24–25
    about fantasies, 170–71
    during intercourse, 132–34
    about likes/needs, 86–88, 115–16, 202
    about oral sex, 86–88
    after sex, 153, 160–61
    tips for, 196–99
complaints, 57–58
condoms, 95
confidence, 25, 200
conversation
    See also communication
    to avoid, 57–59
    seductive, 28–29
criticisms, 57–58, 144–45, 161
cuddling, after sex, 151–52
cunnilingus, 83–90

deep throat technique, 77–78
desires. See fantasies

dirty talk, 44, 59, 145
discomfort, 145
disinterest, 112, 142–43
distractions, 144
doggy style, 121–23
dominance and submission, 187–93
douching, 88

ears, 60, 82
emotional distance, 162
emotional intimacy, 153
emotions, talking about, 17
enjoyment, of sex, 112–13, 199–200
enthusiasm
    lack of, 112, 142–43
    for oral sex, 68–69, 74–75
    for sex, 147, 199
erogenous zones, 27, 50–51, 60–61, 81–83
experimentation, 127–29
    See also fantasies
eye contact, 27–28
eyes, 32

face-to-face positions, 123–24
fantasies, 167–93
    acting out, 171–72
    BDSM, 187–93
    infidelity and, 172–73, 177, 201
    men's views on, 168–74
    about other people, 172–73
    pornography and, 174–81
    role-playing, 183–87
    sharing, 170–71, 198–99
    types of, 173–74
    videotaping sex, 182–83
feedback, 86–88, 116
fellatio. See oral sex
female genitals, 32
    See also cunnilingus
first moves, by women, 23–24, 116–17
flirting, 19, 44
foreplay, 41–63
    to avoid, 54–59
    erogenous zones for, 60–61
    extended, 47
    hottest types of, 48–53

kissing as, 45, 50, 59–60
men's views on, 42–48
mental, 48–49
nonphysical, 44–45
oral sex as, 53
penile stimulation, 47–48
sex talk as, 197
skipping, 46
speaking up about need for, 45–46
forwardness, 56–57
fragrance, 34

genitals
female, 32
male, 47–48, 70

hand jobs, 93–109
lubricants for, 94–95
masturbation, 106–8
men's views on, 94–101
oral sex and, 70–71, 75–77
technique, 95–106
hard-to-get women, 18
honesty, 138
hotels, 130–31
hygiene, 55–56, 88–89, 143–44

ice cubes, 81
infidelity, 172–73, 177, 201
inhibitions, 113
initiative, women taking, 23–24, 116–17
inner thighs, 60, 82
insecurities, 19–20
instructions, giving, during
intercourse, 133–34, 196–97
intercourse, 111–47
communication during, 115–16,
132–34
experimentation in, 127–29
favorite positions for, 119–27
frequency of, 117–18
Kegels for better, 141–42
locations for, 129–32
men's views on, 112–18
orgasms during, 134–38
recharging after, 153–54
time to wait before having, 36–39
turn-offs, 142–46
videotaping, 182–83

Kama Sutra, 128
Kegels, 111–12, 141–42

kinkiness, 187–93
kissing, 45, 50, 59–60

lack of interest, 68–69, 112, 142–43
laughter, 164
living rooms, 131–32
locations, for sex, 104–5, 129–32
lovemaking. See intercourse
lubricants, 94–95, 119

manipulation tactics, 20–21
masturbation, 106–9, 201
men
nice vs. charming, 21–22
orgasms faked by, 136–38
seduction efforts by, 16–22
state of mind of, after sex, 150–51
mental foreplay, 48–49
mirrors, 128
missionary position, 119, 123, 124, 126
mouth, 60
multiple orgasms, 138–41
mutual masturbation, 107, 108
mystery, 22

naked pictures, 182–83
neck, 60, 82
negative attitude, 54–55, 68–69
nice guys, 21–22
nipples, 60, 81
noises, 17, 88, 116, 132–33, 196
nooners, 46

obligatory sex, 112, 142–43
oral sex, 53, 65–90
cunnilingus, 83–90
erogenous zones for, 81–83
men's views on, 66–72
mistakes in performing, 68
rhythm and pressure for, 72–74
technique, 66–68, 70–81
orgasms
faking, 134–38
female, 113, 134–35, 138–39
multiple, 138–41
sequential, 139
simultaneous, 146
truth about, 134–38
outdoors, sex in, 130

penis, 47–48, 70
perineum, 81–82

personal hygiene, 55–56, 88–89, 143–44
personality changes, 163–64
pictures, 182–83
pornography, 174–83
positions, sex, 119–27
    face-to-face, 123–24
    missionary, 119, 123, 124, 126
    rear entry, 121–23
    side-by-side, 126
    standing, 128
    variety in, 125–29
    woman on top, 119–21, 123–24
postcoital period, 149–65
    cuddling during, 151–52
    men's views on, 150–55
    recharging during, 153–54
    sleeping during, 156–60
    state of bliss during, 150–51
    turn-offs during, 160–65
prostate area, 84
prudery, 57
pubic hair, 61–62, 89
public places, sex in, 129

quickies, 46, 152

rear-entry position, 121–23
rejection, 19, 20
relationships
    assumptions about, 161–62
    talking about, 153, 160–61
    time to develop, 36–39
relaxation, 151, 158–59
remorse, 163
rhythm, 67, 72–74, 79, 98–99, 104
role-playing, 183–87
    See also BDSM
rough sex, 187–93

sadomasochism, 187–93
saliva, 71, 95
scrotum, 60
seduction
    dressing for, 34–35
    male efforts at, 16–22
    male insecurity about, 19–20
    secrets of, 15–39
    tips for, 24–29
    by women, 23–29
self-confidence, 146
self-consciousness, 57, 113
self-deprecating remarks, 58

sequential orgasms, 139
sex. See intercourse; oral sex
sex positions. See positions, sex
sexual chemistry, 36–37
sexual daydreams, 168–69
    See also fantasies
sexual fantasies. See fantasies
sexual intercourse.
    See intercourse
sexual interest, signs of male, 16–17
sexual role-playing, 183–87
shoulders, 32
side-by-side position, 126
sleeping, after sex, 151, 152, 154, 156–60
smell, 34, 55–56
smoking, 164
spontaneity, 132
standing positions, 128

talking dirty, 44, 59, 145
teeth, 71, 79–80
testicles, 71, 79, 81
timing, during intercourse, 115–16, 117
tongue techniques, 78–79
touching
    as foreplay, 50–51
    as seduction, 25–27
trust, 21, 190
turn-offs
    during foreplay, 54–59
    for intercourse, 112, 142–46
    in postcoital period, 160–65
    tushes, 29–32, 121–23

variety
    in oral sex, 66–67, 73–74, 75–77
    sexual, 114
    of sexual positions, 125–29
verbal cues, 28–29, 48–49, 132–33
verbal turn-offs, 144–45
videotape, 182–83

waxing, 61–62, 89
woman-on-top position, 119–21, 123–24
women
    first moves by, 23–24, 116–17
    lack of interest by, 112, 142–43
    orgasms by, 113, 134–35, 138–39
    playing hard-to-get, 18
    seduction by, 23–29
    watching masturbate, 107–9